MCQ Tutor in Basic Sciences for Anaesthesia

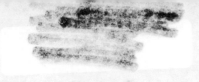

For Churchill Livingstone

Publisher: Simon Fathers
Project Editor: Clare Wood-Allum
Editorial Co-ordination: Editorial Resources Unit
  Copy Editor: Delia Malim-Robinson
Production Controller: Neil Dickson
Design: Design Resources Unit
Sales Promotion Executive: Louise Johnstone

MCQ Tutor in Basic Sciences for Anaesthesia

Colin A. Pinnock
MB BS FRCAnaes
Consultant Anaesthetist, Alexandra Hospital, Redditch, UK

Robert P. Jones
MB ChB DA(UK)
Registrar in Anaesthetics, Alexandra Hospital, Redditch, UK

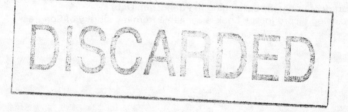

CHURCHILL LIVINGSTONE
EDINBURGH LONDON MADRID MELBOURNE NEW YORK AND TOKYO 1992

CHURCHILL LIVINGSTONE
Medical Division of Longman Group UK Limited

Distributed in the United States of America by Churchill
Livingstone Inc., 650 Avenue of the Americas, New York, N.Y. 10011,
and by associated companies, branches and representatives
throughout the world.

© Longman Group UK Limited 1992

First published 1992

ISBN 0-443-04611-5

British Library Cataloguing in Publication Data
A catalogue record for this book is available from the British Library.

Library of Congress Cataloging in Publication Data
A catalog record for the book is available from the Library of Congress.

The
publisher's
policy is to use
paper manufactured
from sustainable forests

Produced by Longman Singapore Publishers (Pte) Ltd
Printed in Singapore

Preface

This book has been written for two main reasons. The first is to air material which has been extensively used and tested over several years to a wider audience. The second and perhaps more important is to fill a niche in the currently available revision texts for candidates sitting the Part 2 FRCAnaes examination. Good as the existing texts are, this volume attempts something more ambitious. It sets out to reproduce the format and style of question as used in the actual examination. Further, every single answer given has a numerical reference to a source of established expertise.

The pass rate in the Part 2 FRCAnaes currently hovers around 35% and 300 or so candidates sit this examination at each of the two annual sittings. This volume of revision questions is a sincere attempt to help candidates achieve success in this career hurdle.

Whilst previous multiple choice question (MCQ) revision texts have contained discursive answers, this text has gone one step further down that road. A large amount of preparation time has been spent in obtaining references to each answer given so that readers can both satisfy themselves of its validity and, where necessary, read around the topic. Every effort has been made to use standard textbooks for the references. Most anaesthetists in training will have ready access to favourites such as 'Ganong' and 'Synopsis'. On some occasions it has been necessary to delve into more obscure sources. It has been illuminating to find during the construction of this book that the study of one major text in each of the basic sciences is insufficient for revision. Candidates are recommended to use as wide a range of material as possible. A browse through the bibliography at the end of this book may help.

Without doubt it would have been a far easier task to have constructed this volume by writing both question and answer together using common knowledge. This has not been the case. Each question was selected from a variety of sources as being representative of the actual examination. The answers were then sought in published texts and referenced so as to have a basis in fact. It will be apparent to readers that 'correct' responses to MCQ questions are always subject to some dispute. This book attempts to reduce, if not resolve, the ambiguity. Some questions which appear badly worded or ambiguous have been included deliberately. In an ideal world every question asked would be clear and incapable of being misconstrued. In reality candidates will on occasion face ambiguity and the need to make a choice. Several questions in the book raise this very problem and advice is given to the effect that some questions may be best left unanswered. Inevitably in any MCQ text the material may have similarity to other existing works. To the best of my knowledge none of the questions in this book has been obtained from another published work. If similarities exist, as they often do in MCQ revision

Preface

books, I can only apologize for the resemblance, which is not in any way intentional.

I am delighted to applaud the large contribution made to this work by Robert Jones whose enthusiasm and hard work made the idea struggle into reality. I am pleased to acknowledge him as a full co-author of this text.

Finally I am extremely grateful to my colleagues in the Alexandra Hospital for their indulgence and help over the period of writing. My special thanks are due to Dr Peter Scott for his invaluable help with proof reading.

Redditch 1992   C. A. Pinnock

Acknowledgements

There are direct quotes from the following sources:
Question 7, Reference 7.6, Goodman & Gilman
Question 53, Reference 53.7, AHFS
Question 103, Reference 103.3, Recent Advances 16
Question 106, Reference 106.4, Concise Oxford English Dictionary
Question 128, Reference 128.3, Nunn
Question 142, Reference 142.5, Atkinson, Rushman & Lee
Question 189, Reference 189.1, Scurr, Feldman & Soni.

Contents

A Guide to the Part 2 FRCAnaes Examination

THE FRCAnaes DIPLOMA

The three-part examination for the Diploma of Fellow of the Royal College of Anaesthetists is intended to test both depth of knowledge and application of that knowledge across the fields of anaesthesia covered in basic specialist training (BST). In brief these comprise general anaesthetic practice, intensive care medicine, and the relief of chronic pain. The second part of this examination (Part 2 FRCAnaes) tests the basic sciences of pharmacology and physiology relevant to the practice of anaesthesia.

AIMS OF THE PART 2 FRCAnaes

Candidates who achieve success in this section will already have gained a detailed knowledge of basic anaesthetic practice as tested in the Part 1 examination. Success in the second part will demonstrate a sound and thorough grounding in the basic sciences which will enable progress to be made in clinical experience leading to success in the final part of the examination and the attainment of the diploma itself.

THE SCOPE OF THE PART 2 FRCAnaes

PHYSIOLOGY

The principles of basic human physiology. Application of these principles to clinical practice, especially in the fields of artificial ventilation, general anaesthesia, and intensive care medicine. Specialized knowledge of the cardiovascular, respiratory, and neurological systems. The physical principles underlying the measurement of physiological variables with particular emphasis on functional testing of the cardiovascular, respiratory, neurological, renal, and hepatic systems.

PHARMACOLOGY

Basic chemical reactions and the properties of molecules. Physical and chemical properties of therapeutic agents and their formulation. Pharmacokinetics and pharmacodynamics; principles thereof and applications. Drug–receptor interactions and the variability in response of individuals. Detailed pharmacology of those drugs used widely in anaesthetic practice and generalized pharmacological knowledge of other drug groups outside the specialty, particularly those which may be seen frequently as intercurrent medication in patients presenting for surgery. Drug delivery systems. Simple statistics especially with relation to the design and interpretation of clinical trials. Population distributions and their analytical treatment. Estimation of power of a study and confidence limits. Principles of analysing data both parametric and non-parametric including suitable tests for different types of data.

THE STRUCTURE OF THE PART 2 FRCAnaes EXAMINATION

The examination has three sections:
1. MCQ paper. 80 questions of which 40 concern pharmacology and 40 physiology. The time allowed is 160 min.
2. Oral examination in pharmacology with two examiners. The time allowed is 20 min.
3. Oral examination in physiology with two examiners. The time allowed is 20 min.

MARKING SYSTEM

A close marking system is used in all parts of the examination. The system is as follows:
2+ A good pass and very difficult to obtain!
2   A pass.
1+ A bare fail.
1   A bad fail.
The MCQ paper is marked separately for physiology and pharmacology as are the vivas. To achieve success minimum marks of 2, 2, 2 and 1+ are required. Candidates failing the MCQ paper badly (1 in physiology and 1 in pharmacology) are referred for one examination. The oral examination usually follows the MCQ paper by 4 weeks or so.

Detailed information on all parts of the examination is available in the College publication entitled 'Guide to Training', May 1990. This is available on request from The Royal College of Anaesthetists at 48/49 Russell Square, London WC1. Alternatively it can be obtained from local College Tutors.

Notes on MCQ Technique

Multiple choice question papers are designed to test factual recall. Throughout the three parts of the FRCAnaes the same multiple choice format is used. This consists of an interrogative or <u>stem</u> followed by five separate <u>completions</u> which may be marked true, false, or don't know.

Candidates score +1 mark for each correct response and −1 for each incorrect response while don't know scores zero. In the examination a question book is provided in which are the stems and completions and also a lector sheet on which to mark answer choices by way of pencilled bars. It is most strongly advised that answers are made in the question book before transferring them to the lector sheet. At this stage be absolutely scrupulous in marking the lector sheet in accordance with your answers as minor errors in numbering will prove disastrous. It is all too easy under stress to become confused.

Certain pitfalls deserve mention. Double check any question or part relating to opposites, for example hypo and hyper. If you get the sense reversed then minus five marks will result.

Beware of double negatives which needlessly confuse. While ideally there should not be any, in reality you will meet a few at least. Do not be overly suspicious of obvious false distractors. It is tempting to assume that if only you were more widely read then you would know of the connection between serum molybdenum and halothane hepatitis. Readers will be quick to spot that extensive reading is essential as a defence against this situation. Subjects which involve a great deal of controversy and debate may be best avoided for safety but there is an obvious limit to that particular gambit. There are remarkably few MCQ questions which are all true or all false <u>but</u> remember that these may occasionally occur. Be very suspicious of 'always' and 'never' in a stem. It is also difficult to put value judgements on 'frequently' and 'often'.

When MCQ papers are marked by computer, which is the commonest procedure, each of the completions is ascribed a facility index and a discrimination index. Put simply the facility index is the proportion of candidates answering that particular stem correctly. It is an index of 'easiness'.

In contrast the discrimination index provides a measure of how well a particular stem will distinguish between good and bad candidates. This is obtained by choosing a proportion of good and bad candidates (for example the top and bottom 25%) and subtracting the number of correct answers in the lower category from those in the top. Hopefully a positive figure is obtained. In situations where the discrimination index is negative (in other words where more bad than good candidates scored highly) the completion needs examining for poor construction.

Application of these indices will lead to an evolving higher standard of both stem and completion. Regrettably the need for the introduction of new material on a regular basis requires the process to be continuous.

In summary practical points to keep in the front of your mind as you confront the question paper are listed below for emphasis.

MOST IMPORTANT — DO NOT GUESS!

1. READ EACH QUESTION VERY CAREFULLY.
2. MAKE SURE THAT YOU FULLY UNDERSTAND IT.
3. BE ESPECIALLY WARY OF QUESTIONS WITH OPPOSITES.
4. DO NOT SPEND TOO MUCH TIME ON ANY ONE QUESTION.
5. THINK CLEARLY AND DO NOT PANIC.
6. DO NOT PURSUE THE ANSWER TOO FAR BUT RESPOND ONLY TO THE SIMPLE QUESTION WHICH HAS BEEN POSED.
7. LEAVE SUFFICIENT TIME TO COMPLETE THE LECTOR SHEET.

How to Use the Book

The maximum benefit from using this book as a revision aid will be obtained if the basic reading has been completed first. The layout of the book is consistent; the questions are grouped in batches of 40 alternating between pharmacology and physiology. This deliberately mirrors the present examination structure. As you work through the book you will find on the left-hand page two questions each preceded by a short introduction. Below them on the same page are listed the references which are keyed to the answers. Each couplet of questions has the answers displayed on the right-hand page.

It is suggested for revision that a sheet of paper or card is used to cover the answers while the questions are being attempted. Apart from concealing the answers this sheet may be used to record your choices for each completion. If a question is encountered about which you know very little, use the references below to read around the subject before answering. This will make the most of the revision exercise.

The references are quoted in shortened form and most of them will be familiar. A complete list of the short references will be found in the bibliography at the back of the book. They are listed in full in alphabetical order and any unfamiliar source can be identified. Rather than being merely a list the bibliography also gives some weight to the respective relevance of each text. Scanning it will indicate the scope of the reading necessary. Nearly all the texts are the currently available editions. On occasion an earlier edition has been used and where this is so it is specified in the short reference. Some older texts which have not been recently revised have been used where they are classic in nature and likely to be in every postgraduate library. An example of this is Davenport's famous text on acid-base balance (1974).

Finally there is an index of subjects on page 255. Where a topic in the index is followed by a number alone this indicates that the whole question is on that subject. In contrast if a topic is followed by a number and a letter then it is the completion within a question which relates. For example, in the index 'Angiotensin II, 52b, 155' indicates that angiotensin II is featured in question 52, completion b), and is the main subject in question 155 to which all completions will refer.

The index will enable the selection of any one particular topic for revision by indicating each and every occasion on which that topic occurs.

1 Throughout this book you will find a short preamble before each question which relates to the topic and may at times give some factual help. The kind of stem below where each completion involves a different topic makes for a very searching question. While this is efficient from an examiner's point of view it does require knowledge over a very large area. In this particular question there is a mix of completions ranging from the obscure to the obvious; some marks at least should be easy to achieve. Do not guess.

The following associations are found:
a) propranolol and nightmares
b) alpha methyldopa and anaemia
c) phenothiazines and abnormal gait
d) penicillin and convulsions
e) prednisolone and hyperkalaemia

2 Methyl alcohol and ethyl alcohol are not identical compounds although they do share a number of similar pharmacological properties. Poisoning by methyl alcohol (and ethyl alcohol!) is not uncommon. It may be helpful to draw on clinical experience in order to answer this question. If you are confused or achieve low marks use the references to find a text to study and then attempt the question again.

In methyl alcohol toxicity:
a) treatment is ethyl alcohol
b) the methyl alcohol is metabolized to acetaldehyde
c) there may be retrobulbar neuritis
d) there is hyperaemia of the optic disc
e) there is severe metabolic acidosis

References	
1.1 Goodman & Gilman	p 238–239
1.2 BNF	section 2.5.2
1.3 BNF	section 4.2.1
1.4 BNF	section 5.1.1.1
1.5 Goodman & Gilman	p 1441
2.1 Rang & Dale	p 892–893
2.2 Goodman & Gilman	p 1624

1a) T Propranolol has various effects on the central nervous system in common with the beta-blockers in general. The effects include sleep disturbances, especially insomnia and nightmares (1.1). Symptoms may be so marked as to require withdrawal of treatment in some patients. The mechanism is not clear but probably adrenergic balance within the central nervous system is upset.

b) T Alpha methyldopa therapy may be complicated by an autoimmune Coombs positive haemolytic anaemia (1.2). Alpha methyldopa is waning in popularity as a treatment for hypertension but it is not unusual to find patients who have been stabilized on the drug for some years presenting for surgery.

c) T Tardive dyskinesia and Parkinsonian gait occur in patients on phenothiazine medication (1.3). As a group the phenothiazines are renowned for their Parkinsonian side-effects. These can occur with a member of the butyrophenones (which closely resemble group three phenothiazines) used widely in anaesthetic practice, i.e. droperidol.

d) T Penicillin can penetrate the blood–brain barrier. One of the rare but serious toxic effects is the development of encephalopathy which may be complicated by convulsions (1.4). Remember that a number of patients show true allergy to penicillin. Should patients allergic to the drug receive it there is a risk of the development of anaphylaxis. This may lead to cardiovascular collapse with or without convulsions and possibly death.

e) F This is false. An infrequent effect seen during treatment with corticosteroids is hypokalaemic alkalosis which is the opposite (1.5).

2a) T Ethyl alcohol (ethanol) is a recognized form of treatment for cases of methyl alcohol poisoning. The metabolism of methyl alcohol to formaldehyde is retarded by large doses of ethanol because ethanol competes for alcohol dehydrogenase and thus slows down the metabolism of methyl alcohol to toxic metabolites (2.1).

b) F Methyl alcohol (methanol) is metabolized in its first oxidation step to formaldehyde, not acetaldehyde. In contrast, ethyl alcohol is metabolized to acetaldehyde. The metabolic pathway for both these reactions is the same (2.1).

c) F Beware of the casual answer here. It is well known that blindness results from consumption of methyl alcohol. The blindness is due to formation of formaldehyde and formic acid in the retina itself. The enzyme responsible for this process is endogenous dehydrogenase which is normally responsible for retinol conversion (2.1).

d) T Hyperaemia of the optic disc does indeed occur (2.2). This is detectable clinically in some cases by ophthalmoscopy. Clinical experience may help here.

e) T In methyl alcohol poisoning formic acid is produced by metabolism. Formic acid cannot be metabolized in the Krebs cycle as can acetic acid. Thus a severe metabolic acidosis results from derangement of the Krebs cycle and the accumulation of formic acid (2.1).

3 The Digitalis alkaloids are widely prescribed. The elderly population is particularly likely to be treated with these drugs. Patients may have toxic plasma levels of cardiac glycosides when presenting for surgery. Consider that this question could also be phrased to apply to one of the other glycosides, for example ouabain. Is your knowledge of the group adequate?

Overdosage with digoxin:
a) leads to a prolonged P–R interval
b) leads to a prolonged Q–T interval
c) causes diarrhoea
d) can cause xanthopsia
e) is indicated by plasma levels above 1 μg/ml

4 Histamine makes a regular appearance in the examination. Several drugs that are used in anaesthesia cause its release in significant quantities. The development of antagonists to different histamine receptors keeps the topic very much to the fore.

Histamine:
a) belongs to the autacoids
b) has two receptor types, H_1 and H_2
c) causes bronchoconstriction
d) reduces peripheral resistance
e) reduces preload

References

3.1 Goodman & Gilman   p 832–834
3.2 BNF   section 2.1.1

4.1 Vickers, Morgan & Spencer   p 236–239

3a) T Digoxin toxicity typically causes abnormalities of cardiac rhythm and disturbances of atrioventricular (A–V) conduction including complete A–V block. The P–R interval is therefore prolonged in most instances (3.1).

b) F Abnormalities of conduction in the ventricular specialized conducting system and in the ventricles are rarely seen in digoxin toxicity. The Q–T interval will thus remain normal (3.1).

c) T Gastrointestinal effects of toxic levels of digoxin are frequently seen. They include anorexia, nausea, vomiting, diarrhoea, and abdominal discomfort (3.1).

d) T Xanthopsia, or yellow vision, is a frequent complaint in overdosage with cardiac glycosides. Many disturbances of vision can occur with digoxin toxicity. Other changes in colour vision (chromatopsia) include green, red, brown, and blue (3.1).

e) F No single plasma level gives a reliable indication of toxicity but the likelihood increases through the range 1.5–3 µg/l (3.2). Therapeutic levels are seen at less than 1.0 µg/l.

4a) T This term is used to apply to the group of substances which have their effects locally at the site of release. Histamine shares this group with 5-HT (5-hydroxytryptamine) and SRS (slow-releasing substance) amongst others (4.1).

b) T The various receptor subtypes for histamine are well documented. H_2 receptors are involved in acid release from the stomach and some cardiovascular effects whereas H_1 receptors mediate all the other actions of histamine (4.1). Large numbers of patients are receiving H_2 antagonists, most commonly cimetidine and ranitidine.

c) T Bronchoconstriction results from direct stimulation of bronchiolar muscle. It is unrelated to nervous innervation (4.1). The occurrence of severe bronchospasm during anaphylactic reaction will not be readily forgotten once observed.

d) T Peripheral resistance falls due to dilatation of arterioles and capillaries (4.1). A pink flush is often seen after parenteral use of anaesthetic agents which cause histamine release and this is due to the histaminic action on vessels.

e) T The dilatation of capillaries causes stasis with reduced venous return and reduced preload. There is also a rise in cerebrospinal fluid (CSF) pressure which produces an intense and pounding headache (4.1).

5 Acetylsalicylic acid (aspirin) is a drug frequently used without pre-scription as a non-steroidal anti-inflammatory drug (NSAID). It is important to know about this group of drugs and their interactions. Be sure that you have a clear classification of this group before sitting the examination. Do not be surprised to face interrogation on the with-drawn drugs from this group and the reasons for their withdrawal.

Acetylsalicylic acid:
a) is an antipyretic agent
b) affects carbohydrate metabolism
c) may increase uric acid excretion
d) is related to microcytic anaemia
e) can cause dizziness

6 Although infrequently used today the action of hydralazine illustrates several important physiological principles. In the clinical arena hydra-lazine still proves a useful agent to have to hand for the intravenous control of severe acute hypertension.

Hydralazine:
a) exerts its effect via baroreceptor reflexes
b) is a direct vasodilator
c) decreases afterload
d) may lead to SLE syndrome
e) is an alpha-blocker

References

5.1 Vickers, Morgan & Spencer   p 189–193

6.1 Goodman & Gilman   p 799–800
6.2 Drug and Therapeutics Bulletin
     Adverse Drug Reaction Bulletin
     (1987) 123   p 460–463

5a) T This is true although acetylsalicylic acid (aspirin) only has an anti-pyretic effect in pre-existing pyrexial states. This effect is mediated via the hypothalamus. Heat loss is increased due to sweating and hyperaemia of the skin. If sweating fails to occur, for example in electrolyte depletion, then hyperpyrexia will result (5.1).

b) T Large doses of acetylsalicylic acid will paradoxically reduce glycosuria in diabetics. In normal subjects hyperglycaemia and glycosuria both occur (5.1).

c) T There is a paradoxical dose-dependent action of acetylsalicylic acid on the excretion of uric acid. At doses of 1–2 g/24 h net excretion is diminished because active tubular excretion is depressed more than reabsorption. Above 4–5 g/24 h tubular reabsorption dominates with the overall effect being enhanced excretion (5.1).

d) T Gastric erosions are common and chronic bleeding occurs in about 80% of patients taking more than 4 g/24 h. Usual blood losses are 3–10 ml/24 h although sometimes there is sufficient bleeding to cause an iron deficiency anaemia (5.1). Enteric coated versions of aspirin have been produced in an attempt to minimize this problem. Usually advice is given to patients to avoid taking the drug on an empty stomach.

e) T Dizziness, especially combined with tinnitus, is common with large or repeated doses of acetylsalicylic acid (5.1). Both symptoms can occur in cases of poisoning. The clinical picture may be clouded by the common practice of mixing drugs for deliberate overdosage. A mixture of aspirin and alcohol is one example where dizziness is a certainty.

6a) F The effect of hydralazine is primarily a direct action on arteriolar smooth muscle. The mechanism of this effect is not clear (6.1). This is a dangerous question to answer. There is activation of the baro-receptors as a reflex response to the hypotensive effect of the drug. The degree of the response is related to the initial tone of the baro-receptor system prior to administration of hydralazine.

b) T Hydralazine causes a preferential dilatation of arterioles over veins and a selective decrease in vascular resistance in the coronary, cerebral, and renal circulation with a smaller effect in skin and muscle (6.1).

c) T The reduction in afterload follows from the preferential arteriolar dilatation. There is an increase in cardiac output but this is due to a baroreceptor mediated reflex (6.1).

d) T This is a well known association. The incidence of lupus syndrome is related to dose, sex, acetylator phenotype, and race (6.1). Systemic lupus erythematosus (SLE) syndrome is characterized by a delayed onset of 1 month to 5 years. The clinical manifestations include poly-arthritis, fever, myalgia, and various pulmonary features. Pericar-ditis is common and skin rashes may occur (6.2).

e) F Hydralazine has no alpha blocking activity. Its action is confined to vascular smooth muscle relaxation (6.1).

7 It is vital in any MCQ examination to understand the stem and to know the meaning of all words used therein. An error in your reading or understanding of the stem could result in a subtraction of five marks. Mydriasis is the technical word for pupillary dilatation (7.1) while miosis describes pupillary constriction. During revision it will be useful to spend some time studying the nerve supply of the eye and the effects of drugs on pupil size.

The following drugs cause mydriasis:
a) cocaine
b) neostigmine
c) guanethidine
d) imipramine
e) cyclopentolate

8 Acetazolamide is occasionally used in anaesthesia and intensive care. It is important both historically and in context of the examination because of its action on carbonic anhydrase. During ophthalmic surgery intravenous administration of the drug may be requested by the surgeon. It behoves all of us to have a thorough understanding of any agent to which we subject a patient.

Acetazolamide:
a) can cause metabolic acidosis
b) raises intraocular pressure
c) can be taken orally
d) is a carbonic anhydrase inhibitor
e) is a pupillary dilator

References	
7.1 Vickers, Morgan & Spencer	p 295
7.2 Goodman & Gilman	p 319
7.3 Vickers, Morgan & Spencer	p 288
7.4 BNF	section 11.6
7.5 Data Sheet Compendium	p 1609
7.6 Goodman & Gilman, 5th edn	p 175
7.7 Goodman & Gilman	p 405–413
7.8 Rang & Dale	p 154–156
8.1 Goodman & Gilman	p 716
8.2 BNF	section 11.6
8.3 Rang & Dale	p 422

7a) T Cocaine dilates the pupil by adrenergic stimulation. Cocaine blocks the uptake of catecholamines at adrenergic nerve endings. It is uptake of catecholamines which is the principal mechanism responsible for the termination of the actions of both adrenergic nervous impulses and circulating catecholamines (7.2).

b) F The anticholinesterases all cause miosis (7.3). Physostigmine eye drops can be used as a long-acting miotic in the treatment of glaucoma (7.4).

c) T Beware! Guanethidine when used alone as eye drops produces initial mydriasis followed by miosis (7.5). Therefore the answer to this question is true; however, some authorities dispute the initial mydriatic action. Because of the doubt and the possibility of not remembering the facts correctly in the stressful examination situation it might be better to answer 'don't know'.

d) F In the list of side-effects of tricyclic antidepressants most sources quote anticholinergic effects including blurring of vision and then omit to state any effect on the pupil. An early edition of a standard text states 'There is little, if any change in pupillary size' (7.6). This statement refers to a single oral dose of 100 mg imipramine and is not found in the most recent edition (7.7).

e) T Deliberately developed for mydriasis, cyclopentolate has a shorter action than atropine when used as eye drops prior to ophthalmoscopic examination. The effects of atropine eye drops last for several days, usually to the patient's chagrin (7.8).

8a) T The concentration of bicarbonate in extracellular fluid falls as a direct effect of the inhibition of carbonic anhydrase and increased urinary excretion of bicarbonate. Metabolic acidosis results (8.1). This will not usually be a feature in short-term treatment.

b) F The carbonic anhydrase present in the eye is inhibited and so the bicarbonate in aqueous humour is reduced. Water is normally secreted together with the bicarbonate and thus intraocular pressure falls (8.2).

c) T There are currently available preparations of acetazolamide for administration by the oral, intravenous, and intramuscular routes (8.2).

d) T A potent reversible inhibition of carbonic anhydrase occurs at several sites. In the kidney this causes a diuresis and in the eye a reduction in intraocular pressure. Inhibition may occur in the pancreas and gastric mucosa too (8.3).

e) F Acetazolamide reduces the rate of <u>formation</u> of aqueous humour and has no effect on pupil size or drainage of aqueous humour (8.3).

9 Diazoxide is one of the more interesting vasoactive agents because it has diverse effects on several organ systems. Although the drug is not commonly met in modern practice you can expect to meet it on occasion in examinations.

Diazoxide:
a) is an antihypertensive agent
b) causes hypoglycaemia
c) causes hypocalcaemia
d) is usually given intravenously
e) is a vasodilator

10 In an anaesthesia diploma examination there will naturally be questions on anaesthetic agents. It is expected that you will know in detail those drugs which are used in everyday practice. Most hospitals in the UK will have a methohexitone user in the theatre suite although the popularity of this agent is waning.

Methohexitone:
a) is excreted unchanged in the urine
b) has four isomers
c) is a thiobarbiturate
d) may cause pain on injection
e) has a pH of 11

References
9.1 Goodman & Gilman   p 804–805
9.2 Vickers, Morgan & Spencer p 346–348

10.1 Goodman & Gilman   p 1690
10.2 Atkinson, Rushman & Lee   p 236–237
10.3 Vickers, Morgan & Spencer p 65
10.4 Aitkenhead & Smith   p 177–178
10.5 Dundee & Wyant   ch 5

9a) T A profound dilatation of arteriolar smooth muscle occurs with very little effect on the capacitance vessels. Diazoxide hyperpolarizes arterial smooth muscle cells by activating adenosine triphosphate (ATP)-sensitive K^+ channels and so causing relaxation (9.1).

b) F Hyperglycaemia occurs in at least 50% of patients taking the drug (9.1). It is due to a rise in circulatory catecholamine levels and a direct inhibitory action on the beta cells of the pancreas to block insulin release (9.2). This is not surprising given the close resemblance in structure of the drug to the thiazide family.

c) F Diazoxide does not cause hypocalcaemia. Note, however, that there is some interference with calcium receptors or bound intracellular calcium at a cellular level (9.2).

d) T Originally diazoxide was marketed as an oral preparation but had unacceptable side-effects, particularly hyperglycaemia. Later it was marketed as an intravenous preparation for treatment of hypertensive emergencies. Sodium nitroprusside then appeared on the scene and has largely usurped this role (9.1).

e) T Sometimes this completion may be phrased 'is a venodilator'. The effect of the drug is exclusively arteriolar (9.1). Read stems and completions meticulously before answering.

10a) F Less than 1% of methohexitone is excreted in the urine unchanged or changed (10.1). (Reference 10.1 is a very comprehensive table of pharmacokinetic data which have previously been difficult to obtain).

b) T Methohexitone occurs in four different isomers because of its two asymmetric carbon atoms. There are two pairs of isomers: alpha D and L forms and beta D and L forms. The alpha pair have less effect on skeletal muscle tone and it is these that are present in the commercial preparation (10.2).

c) F Thiopentone is now the only thiobarbiturate in clinical use (10.3). It is important to understand the basis for the names and structures of the barbiturates. A simple table can be used (10.4). For a fuller explanation a more extensive text should be consulted (10.5). The derivations of the clinically used compounds and their relationship to malonic acid may form a part of the viva examination.

d) T Intravenous injection of methohexitone is prone to cause pain on injection (10.2). Some users believe that there is less pain if the solution is made up with saline rather than water.

e) T When used in a 1% solution (i.e. in accordance with common practice) the pH of methohexitone is 11.1 (10.2).

11 Here is a stem concerning a drug which is met in everyday practice. Is your knowledge adequate? If your score is less than three on this one then you will have to work very hard. It is a sobering thought that even an ubiquitous intravenous anaesthetic agent such as thiopentone can reveal a certain embarassing ignorance.

Thiopentone sodium:
a) is unstable in solution
b) contains sulphur
c) is strongly protein bound
d) is excreted in 2 h
e) is a weak base

12 Dantrolene is used in cases of malignant hyperpyrexia or in patients suspected of having susceptibility to the condition. As its use may be at short notice it is important to know about the drug without resorting to textbooks. Incidentally, it is also useful to know where the stocks are held in your hospital and how to gain access to them.

Dantrolene:
a) has been used as a respiratory stimulant
b) is only used in the treatment of malignant hyperpyrexia
c) antagonizes non-depolarizing block
d) relaxes skeletal muscle
e) is supplied mixed with mannitol

References
11.1 Atkinson, Rushman & Lee   p 229–231
11.2 Trissel   p 727
11.3 Goodman & Gilman   p 1710
11.4 Vickers, Morgan & Spencer   p 17

12.1 Goodman & Gilman   p 480–481
12.2 Data Sheet Compendium   p 1018
12.3 Vickers, Morgan & Spencer   p 265

11a) T Sodium thiopentone is soluble in water and alcohol. Anhydrous sodium carbonate is added to prevent formation of free acid by carbon dioxide from the atmosphere. In solution thiopentone is not very stable but can be left for 24–48 h or longer without harm occurring on subsequent injection. A cloudy solution should not be used (11.1). If you need more information there are extensive texts to study (11.2).

b) T Sodium thiopentone is the sulphur analogue of pentobarbitone and has an odour resembling hydrogen sulphide (11.1). The taste of garlic on administration is remarked upon by some patients and this has been postulated to be linked to the sulphur content.

c) T Approximately 70% of thiopentone in the peripheral blood is protein bound (mainly to albumin). The bound fraction is not active but the ratio of bound to unbound form can change. Changes in pH affect binding. Maximum binding occurs at pH 8. Thiopentone concentrations per se can change binding: maximum binding occurs at low plasma concentrations (11.1).

d) F Between 10 and 15% of the drug is metabolized each hour (11.1). Its half-life is 9 h ± 1.6 h. This figure is increased by age (in females only!), cirrhosis of the liver, obesity, and also in neonates (11.3).

e) F Thiopentone is an acid when in electrolyte form in solution. Its pKa is, however, 7.6 (11.4). The pKa of a drug is the dissociation constant and represents the pH value at which the drug is 50% ionized.

12a) F The effects of dantrolene on the central nervous system (CNS) are generally depressant (12.1). Furthermore caution is advised in patients with poor respiratory function (12.2).

b) F Dantrolene plays a 'unique' role in the treatment of malignant hyperpyrexia (12.1). There have been other reported applications for the drug. These include the prevention of suxamethonium pains and the treatment of spasticity.

c) F Dantrolene uncouples excitation–contraction coupling in muscle by interfering with release of ionic calcium from the sarcoplasmic reticulum. Dantrolene has no action on neuromuscular transmission, the membrane action potential, or muscle excitability (12.3).

d) T Dantrolene is sometimes used as a treatment for skeletal muscle spasticity (12.1). Other agents which have been used include baclofen which is featured later in the book.

e) T There are 20 mg dantrolene in a vial together with 3 g mannitol and sufficient sodium hydroxide to yield a pH of 9.5 when reconstituted with 60 ml of water (12.2).

13 The emphasis now shifts to volatile anaesthetic agents. Often the format of such questions involves completions which invite comparisons between different volatile agents. Although the stem below concerns enflurane, two completions require knowledge of halothane so knowledge of volatile agents should be comprehensive.

Enflurane:
a) is an ether
b) has a boiling point within 5°C of halothane
c) is more potent than halothane
d) has convulsant activity
e) is metabolized to fluoride ions

14 Atropine is commonplace in anaesthetic practice and yet its properties are often ignored, perhaps because it is most frequently used in combination with neostigmine at the end of cases. The applied pharmacology of cholinergic and anticholinergic drugs is a veritable minefield for the unwary.

Atropine:
a) is an isomer of hyoscine
b) crosses the blood–brain barrier
c) reduces sweating
d) increases dead space
e) increases FRC

References
13.1 Vickers, Morgan & Spencer — p 142–144
13.2 Dunnill & Colvin — p 8
13.3 Vickers, Morgan & Spencer — p 36–37

14.1 Goodman & Gilman — p 151–153
14.2 Vickers, Morgan & Spencer — p 293–294
14.3 Atkinson, Rushman & Lee — p 139
14.4 Vickers, Morgan & Spencer — p 295–297
14.5 Goodman & Gilman, 5th edn — p 518

13a) T Enflurane is a halogenated ethyl–methyl ether and isoflurane is an isomer of enflurane (13.1). Questions on the structure of the inhalational agents are common. Be prepared to draw the structure of the 'Big Three' on paper.

b) F The boiling point of halothane is 50°F and of enflurane 56°F (13.2). Be careful. Many texts contain tables of the physical properties of volatile agents and the figures often vary. During revision choose one table and don't chop and change as this will lead to confusion. Try learning one volatile agent or one specific property at any one time and cross-referencing them during spare moments when you think that you know the vital statistics. This may prove easier than memorizing a 'railway timetable' at one sitting. These facts are essential.

c) F Potency of volatile agents is related to minimum alveolar concentration (MAC) (13.3). MAC values are approximately: halothane 0.8% v/v, enflurane 1.7% v/v (13.2). Therefore halothane is more potent than enflurane.

d) T In this respect enflurane is different from all other volatile agents producing marked central stimulant actions. The electroencephalogram (EEG) commonly shows episodes of paroxysmal activity and periods of burst suppression. These changes are a function of anaesthetic depth and are exacerbated by a reduction in Pco_2. Episodes of tonic or clonic twitching of the jaws have been observed. The EEG effects may persist for up to 30 *days* after the drug is used and convulsions may occur for up to 7 days after administration. In normocapnic patients enflurane does not worsen pre-existing epilepsy (13.1).

e) T Inorganic fluoride is the major metabolic product. The levels are related to inspired enflurane level and duration of exposure. Maximum serum fluoride levels may reach 25 µmol/l, at which point there may be a reduction in maximum urine concentrating ability. However, in a well-hydrated patient with normal renal function, these effects are of little clinical importance (13.1).

14a) F The structures of atropine and hyoscine (scopolamine) differ (14.1). However, atropine is a racemate (DL-hyoscyamine). It is the L, or laevoisomer, which is most active. Hyoscine is also racemic (14.2).

b) T Since in therapeutic doses atropine causes mild vagal excitation effects as a result of stimulation of the medulla and higher cerebral centres, it must be able to cross the blood–brain barrier (14.1). Some of the effects of atropine poisoning are mediated through central effects.

c) T Atropine is an antagonist of muscarinic receptors. This leads to an inhibition of sweating which may contribute to pyrexia (14.3).

d) T Anatomical dead space is increased due to dilatation of the smooth muscle of the bronchioles (14.4). Note that physiological dead space is also increased but blood gas tensions do not change.

e) T Functional residual capacity (FRC) includes air contained in the bronchioles which are dilated by atropine. FRC will thus increase (14.5).

15 Changes in cerebrovascular resistance (and therefore cerebral blood flow) caused by anaesthetic agents are important on many occasions. Some clinical experience of neuroanaesthesia will prove useful.

The following decrease cerebrovascular resistance:
a) ether
b) isoflurane
c) halothane
d) ketamine
e) thiopentone

16 Salbutamol will be familiar as an agent of value in the treatment of respiratory pathology. In MCQ completions there are often comparisons with older and less frequently used drugs.

With respect to salbutamol:
a) there is more tachycardia than with isoprenaline
b) isoprenaline has a longer duration
c) the effect is mediated through beta$_1$ receptors
d) the intravenous route is faster than the nebulized route
e) tremor may be a problem in some patients

References

15.1 Atkinson, Rushman & Lee	p 179
15.2 Atkinson, Rushman & Lee	p 193
15.3 Atkinson, Rushman & Lee	p 186
16.1 Vickers, Morgan & Spencer	p 247–248
16.2 Rang & Dale	p 204

15a) T Ether will generally increase cerebral blood flow due to vaso-dilatation. CSF pressure will also increase. There will be a decrease in cerebrovascular resistance which parallels the vasodilatation (15.1).

b) T At low inspired concentrations of isoflurane there is no change in cerebral blood flow provided that normocapnia is maintained. With higher inspired concentrations cerebral blood flow does actually show an increase (15.2).

c) T Cerebral blood flow rises as does CSF pressure. Cerebrovascular resistance therefore falls (15.3). Similar changes are seen with most volatile agents.

d) T When ketamine is administered there will be an increase in cerebral blood flow and intracranial pressure although there may be marked regional variations in this respect (15.4).

e) F Thiopentone reduces cerebral blood flow, cerebral metabolism and intracranial pressure (15.5). Thiopentone has applications in intensive care units in cases of severe head injury, both because of these effects and its ability to reduce the cerebral metabolic rate of oxygen consumption ($CMRo_2$).

16a) F The tachycardia seen following the administration of salbutamol is less than that after equipotent doses of isoprenaline (16.1). This is one of the quoted advantages of the drug.

b) F The duration of both agents is dissimilar as can be seen from their half lives. The half life for isoprenaline is approximately 2 h whereas the corresponding half life for salbutamol is 4 h (16.2).

c) F There is little or no effect at $beta_1$ receptors. Salbutamol is a selective $beta_2$ agonist (16.1).

d) F The inhaled route compared with the intravenous produces an immediate effect with marked selectivity for the bronchial tree (16.1). The inhaled route therefore has some advantage in acute situations.

e) T Tremor is common during treatment with salbutamol (16.2). In general this effect is dose dependent.

$t_{1/2}$ isoprenaline 2hr

salbutamol 4hr

17 Questions on benzodiazepine drugs are encountered frequently. They are exceedingly widely prescribed. In general most benzodiazepines share useful actions of hypnosis and anxiolysis. It is principally their various half-lives and metabolites which distinguish them from a practical point of view as premedication agents.

Diazepam:
a) affects the limbic system
b) has a half-life of 20 h
c) is metabolized to oxazepam
d) has anticonvulsant activity
e) affects GABA transmission

18 Although this stem concerns curare the completions are applicable to all non-depolarizing muscle relaxants. While most of this group are familiar, some knowledge of newer agents would be advantageous. Examples of these are doxacurium and mivacurium.

The following potentiate curare:
a) reduced P_{CO_2}
b) metabolic acidosis
c) hypokalaemia
d) hypocalcaemia
e) hypomagnesaemia

References

17.1	Atkinson, Rushman & Lee	p 240
17.2	Rang & Dale	p 635
17.3	Calvey & Williams	p 395
17.4	Calvey & Williams	p 388–391
18.1	Vickers, Morgan & Spencer	p 260–261
18.2	Atkinson, Rushman & Lee	p 260
18.3	Atkinson, Rushman & Lee	p 282

17a) T Benzodiazepines exert their effects via the limbic system and amygdala where fear, anxiety, and aggression are generated. The cerebral cortex is not depressed (17.1). The anxiolytic effect is relevant in premedication.

b) F Although figures vary, most values for the half-life of diazepam exceed 30 h (17.2). It is important to note that an active metabolite of diazepam (nordiazepam or N-desmethyldiazepam) has an average half-life of 60 h with a range of 40–200 h. Diazepam is not a short-acting drug.

c) T Diazepam is demethylated to nordiazepam and thence further hydroxylated to oxazepam. Oxazepam itself has a half-life of 8 h (17.2).

d) T Diazepam is often quoted as the drug of choice in status epilepticus (17.3). Professionally speaking we may consider barbiturates superior in this respect.

e) T Release of the inhibitory neurotransmitter gamma aminobutyric acid (GABA) may be facilitated by benzodiazepines in general (17.4).

18a) T Hyperventilation will lead to hypocapnia and a respiratory alkalosis. Both hypocapnia and alkalosis will prolong apnoea and respiratory depression. This will produce an apparent potentiation of the effect of muscle relaxants (18.1).

b) T Acidosis increases both duration and degree of blockade from curare (18.2). It should be noted that it is only gallamine that is actually antagonized by acidosis. This safety margin has been obscured by the other undesirable features of gallamine, notably its renal excretion and propensity to cause tachycardia.

c) T Hypokalaemia causes increased sensitivity to non-depolarizing relaxants as a whole. It is a relative fall in the ratio of extracellular potassium compared with intracellular potassium that is important. The cell membrane becomes hyperpolarized, there is resistance to the action of acetylcholine, the action of non-depolarizing relaxants is potentiated and that of depolarizing relaxants is antagonized. The response to neostigmine is largely unchanged (18.3).

d) T Hypocalcaemia and hyponatraemia increase sensitivity to non-depolarizing muscle relaxants (18.3).

e) F It is hypermagnesaemia that will potentiate the effect of curare. The effects of calcium and magnesium are opposites here as they are in many physiological applications (18.3).

19 Questions on drug structure and compatibility can be exceedingly searching. To answer such questions reference has frequently been made to Trissel's 'Handbook on Injectable Drugs'. This amazing text is a summary of all of the primary published literature on drug stability and compatibility. Pharmacies will usually have a copy.

A change in pH may alter the structure of the following:
a) suxamethonium
b) tubocurare
c) atracurium
d) midazolam
e) diazepam

20 Motion sickness and drug-induced sickness do not necessarily respond to the same agents although some drugs can be used to treat both conditions. To separate the two mechanisms an understanding of the physiology of emesis is necessary.

The following drugs can reduce motion sickness:
a) metoclopramide
b) imipramine
c) cyclizine
d) domperidone
e) hyoscine

References	
19.1 Trissel	p 711–714
19.2 Trissel	p 755–766
19.3 Trissel	p 76
19.4 Miller	p 245
19.5 Trissel	p 521
19.6 Trissel	p 256
20.1 Rang & Dale	p 456–459

19a) T The pH of maximum stability for suxamethonium is 3.75–4.50. It is rapidly destroyed by alkalization and decomposes in solutions with a pH greater than 4.5. When combined with barbiturates, either free barbituric acid will precipitate or the suxamethonium will be hydrolysed depending on the final pH of the admixture (19.1). Suxamethonium is also temperature sensitive. In tropical climates it is supplied in dry powder form for reconstitution to avoid the necessity for refrigerated storage.

b) T Changes in pH around physiological levels have been cited to cause the curare molecule to change from monoquaternary to bisquaternary. Note also that curare is precipitated from aqueous solution by alkalization (19.2).

c) T A high pH will result in the inactivation of atracurium by Hoffmann elimination. Atracurium is acidic and mixture with alkali will cause inactivation and precipitation of a free acid of the admixed drug. Atracurium is unstable in both acids and bases (19.3).

d) T The imidazole ring structure of the molecule changes in spatial structure with alterations in pH (19.4). Midazolam is stable at pH 3.0–3.6. It is highly water soluble at pH 4 or less. As pH increases lipid solubility increases and the structure changes (19.5).

e) T Diazepam is most stable at pH 4–8 and is subject to acid-catalysed hydrolysis below pH 3 (19.6).

20a) F Metoclopramide is a dopamine receptor antagonist which acts at the chemoreceptor trigger zone. It is used in treatment of sickness associated with uraemia, radiation, and gastrointestinal disorders. Metoclopramide is ineffective in motion sickness and vomiting from disorders of the labyrinth (20.1).

b) F Although imipramine is a tricyclic antidepressant with anticholinergic side-effects, it would be of no use for acute motion sickness! However, nortriptyline and amitriptyline have significant anticholinergic actions and are H_1 receptor antagonists. These drugs are effective against emetogenic cytotoxic agents when combined with fluphenazine (20.1).

c) T Cyclizine and other H_1 antihistamines are effective in reducing motion sickness possibly by blocking impulses from the labyrinths and from afferent visceral pathways passing to the vomiting centre (20.1).

d) F In general, domperidone, a dopamine receptor antagonist like metoclopramide, acts on the chemoreceptor trigger zone and is unlikely to relieve motion sickness. It is, however, effective in chemotherapy-induced emesis (20.1).

e) T Hyoscine is the most efficacious and is the drug of choice. There are muscarinic receptors in the lateral vestibular nucleus, the nucleus of the tractus solitarius, and on the nucleus ambiguus of the vomiting centre on which the drug acts (20.1). Preparations of hyoscine abound in high street chemists.

21 Metoclopramide is used as an antiemetic and to increase the rate of gastric emptying in anaesthetic practice. In common with every drug metoclopramide is not without unwanted effects. Some of these may prove to be distressing in the extreme.

The following are side-effects of metoclopramide:
a) hypertension
b) oculogyric crisis
c) nausea
d) increased prolactin secretion
e) gynaecomastia

22 Propranolol enjoyed a vogue as a premedicant and some MCQ questions may originate from this era. Nonetheless propranolol and the newer beta-blocking agent derivatives are frequently used as treatments for hypertension and many patients present for surgery receiving such drugs.

Propranolol:
a) may mask hypoglycaemia
b) increases cardiac irritability
c) causes bronchospasm
d) causes tachycardia
e) may be given orally

References
21.1 Data Sheet Compendium   p 148–151
21.2 Goodman & Gilman   p 927
21.3 Meyler's Side Effects   p 783

22.1 Goodman & Gilman   p 229–234

21a) F In the normal adult there is no hypertension but an acute hypertensive crisis may occur in the presence of phaeochromocytoma (21.1) which is an infrequently met condition.

b) T A number of extrapyramidal reactions can occur. These are usually of the dystonic type such as spasm of the facial muscles, trismus, rhythmic protrusion of the tongue, a bulbar type of speech, spasm of extraocular muscles including oculogyric crises, unnatural positioning of the head and shoulders, and opisthotonos (21.1). Many are both painful and distressing. Metoclopramide is not an 'innocuous' anti- emetic.

c) F The drug is frequently used to treat nausea and vomiting in the post-operative period (21.1).

d) T Prolactin secretion is increased by metoclopramide. Hyperprolactinaemia can lead to galactorrhoea, breast tenderness, and menstrual irregularities (21.2).

e) T Gynaecomastia is a recognized effect secondary to hyperprolactinaemia (21.3).

22a) T All beta-blockers mask the tachycardia that is typically seen in hypoglycaemia. Diabetic patients often find tachycardia a useful sign of impending hypoglycaemia (22.1).

b) F Propranolol reduces cardiac irritability and this is part of its antiarrhythmic effect (22.1).

c) T Beta adrenergic antagonists block $beta_2$ adrenergic receptors in bronchial smooth muscle. In normal patients that would cause no problem but in patients with asthma or chronic obstructive pulmonary disease, this blockade can lead to life-threatening bronchoconstriction (22.1).

d) F Beta adrenergic antagonists slow the heart rate and decrease myocardial contractility (22.1). They are thus negative inotropes although in some compounds the effect is offset by a variable degree of intrinsic sympathetic activity (ISA).

e) T There is an oral preparation of propranolol. The large difference in bioavailability between oral and intravenous doses is due to the first pass phenomenon. Following absorption from the gastrointestinal tract the larger proportion of the dose is metabolized by the liver. On average only about 25% of the oral dose reaches the systemic circulation (22.1).

23 It is common to anaesthetize pregnant patients at various stages of pregnancy and it is therefore important to know how the uterus is affected by the drugs that are used. Also anaesthetists encounter patients who are receiving drugs used to influence the uterine tone and it is thus relevant to have knowledge of these agents as well.

The following drugs are uterine relaxants:
a) halothane
b) enflurane
c) atropine
d) salbutamol
e) ritodrine

24 Frusemide is probably the most widely used diuretic. As diuretics are a very common topic in this examination be sure you have a sound enough factual basis to answer on the foremost member of the group.

Frusemide may cause:
a) hypokalaemia
b) hypoglycaemia
c) raised serum urate
d) increased renal blood flow
e) deafness

References	
23.1 Vickers, Morgan & Spencer	p 132
23.2 Goodman & Gilman	p 156
23.3 Vickers, Morgan & Spencer	p 402–407
23.4 BNF	section 7.1.2
24.1 BNF	section 2.2.2
24.2 Goodman & Gilman	p 722–724

23a) T Halothane and chloroform cause relaxation of uterine muscle to such an extent as to make their use unsuitable when sustained uterine activity is desirable (23.1).

b) T Although enflurane relaxes uterine muscle, this effect is not seen in light levels of anaesthesia. This profile also applies to trichloro-ethylene (23.1).

c) F Uterine smooth muscle is innervated by parasympathetic fibres but the effect of cholinergic impulses on contractility is variable. As a result atropine has negligible effects on the human uterus (23.2).

d) T Beta$_2$ adrenergic agonists are uterine relaxants (23.3). Their use in premature labour has led to the popularity of ritodrine for this indication.

e) T Any beta$_2$ agonist can be used to relax the uterus but ritodrine has become the drug of choice in premature labour due to its relative specificity for the uterus. (23.4).

24a) T Hypokalaemia is a secondary effect of potassium loss during the diuresis and hence entirely predictable (24.1).

b) F In contrast, a side-effect of frusemide is hyperglycaemia although this is uncommon (24.1).

c) T Hyperuricaemia is frequently seen and may lead to clinical gout (24.1).

d) T There is a short-lived increase in renal blood flow without an increase in filtration rate, especially after intravenous injection. The change in renal haemodynamics reduces fluid and electrolyte reabsorption in the proximal tubule and may augment the initial diuretic response (24.2).

e) T Deafness may occur during treatment with frusemide. It may be more frequent with higher dose regimens. A disturbance of the ionic composition of endolymph in the cochlea is thought to be a possible mechanism (24.2).

25 Many drugs change the rate of gastric emptying. The completions below include some agents which are deliberately used for their effects on gastric motility. The physiology of the cholinergic system provides the answer with respect to the last two.

The rate of gastric emptying is increased by:
a) metoclopramide
b) ranitidine
c) omeprazole
d) atropine
e) neostigmine

26 The correct answers for most of the completions below are fairly clear cut. The final completion may, however, provoke debate. In an MCQ examination there is no opportunity to debate with the computer that marks the answer papers. The choice of the answer to this completion may rely more on semantics than knowledge.

The following have anticonvulsant activity:
a) phenytoin
b) dantrolene
c) clobazam
d) chlorpromazine
e) bupivacaine

References	
25.1 Rang & Dale	p 458
25.2 Drugs (1989) 37	p 814–816
25.3 Goodman & Gilman	p 903
25.4 BJA (1990) 65	p 607–608
25.5 Goodman & Gilman	p 156
25.6 Goodman & Gilman	p 137
26.1 BNF	section 4.8.1
26.2 Goodman & Gilman	p 480
26.3 BNF	section 4.1.2
26.4 Goodman & Gilman	p 390
26.5 BNF	section 15.2

25a) T Metoclopramide has central antiemetic effects and exerts a local stimulant effect on gastric motility with a marked acceleration of gastric emptying but no concomitant increase in acid secretion (25.1). The use of metoclopramide in accelerating gastric emptying prior to anaesthesia should be reserved for the intravenous route of administration.

b) F Neither cimetidine nor ranitidine increases the rate of gastric emptying. Ranitidine has been shown to delay gastric emptying after a single oral dose of 300 mg in volunteers but this is not an important clinical effect (25.2).

c) F Omeprazole reduces gastric acid secretion but has no effect on gastric emptying (25.3). One of a new group of drugs which inhibit the proton pump, omeprazole is currently gaining ground in the treatment and prevention of peptic ulceration (25.4).

d) F If atropine is given in full therapeutic doses there are prolonged inhibitory effects on the motor activity of the stomach, duodenum, jejunum, ileum, and colon. There is a reduction in tone, amplitude, and frequency of peristaltic contractions. Atropine can effectively block the excess motor activity of the gastrointestinal tract caused by anticholinesterase agents (25.5).

e) T Neostigmine enhances gastric contractility and increases the secretion of gastric acid, its effects being reversed by atropine (25.6).

26a) T Phenytoin is a commonly used agent in the treatment of epilepsy, being recommended for all forms of epilepsy except absence seizures (26.1).

b) T Dantrolene possesses general CNS depressant activity although it has no recommended therapeutic use as an anticonvulsant (26.2).

c) T All benzodiazepines have antiepileptic activity to varying degrees. Clobazam can be used as an 'adjunct' in epilepsy (26.3) but is unlikely to be an agent of first choice.

d) F Like many neuroleptic drugs chlorpromazine lowers the seizure threshold and induces discharge patterns in the EEG that are associated with epileptic convulsions (26.4).

e) F Although local anaesthetic agents are generally membrane stabilizers, the possible CNS effects of a suitable dose for use in anaesthesia are excitation, nausea, and convulsions. Ultimately CNS depression results. Caution is recommended in patients with epilepsy (26.5). The correct answer to this completion is 'false' for although there may be a degree of theoretical antiseizure effect, no one in their right mind would consider a local anaesthetic agent with a narrow therapeutic index for such a role. The moral here would appear to be 'trust the examiner'.

---

27 Questions on opioid drugs may involve named agents or the receptor system. Knowledge of this area should be extensive (27.1, 27.2, 27.3). As the field is expanding so fast it is recommended that current journals are included in revision reading. Candidates should have ready access to the two major UK journals (BJA and Anaesthesia).

Pentazocine:
a) is more potent than morphine
b) is reversed by naloxone
c) can cause hallucinations
d) is a partial agonist
e) binds to kappa receptors

28 Lignocaine is probably the most frequently occurring local anaesthetic agent in the MCQ paper. Remember that there are several other local anaesthetic agents. Questions on this topic may be more generalized than the one below.

Lignocaine:
a) is a vasodilator
b) is metabolized in the liver
c) is an amide
d) has a pKa of 7
e) is a weak base

References

27.1 Current Anaesthesia and
 Critical Care (1990) 1.4   p 252–257
27.2 Anaesthesia Review 3   p 36–62
27.3 BJA (1991) 66   p 370–380
27.4 Rang & Dale   p 718–719
27.5 Rang & Dale   p 729
27.6 Science Data Book   p 87

28.1 Vickers, Morgan & Spencer   p 211–213
28.2 Goodman & Gilman   p 320
28.3 Dundee, Clarke & McCaughey   p 287
28.4 Goodman & Gilman   p 316

27a) F By definition agonist–antagonist drugs are less potent than agonists (27.4). In low doses the effects of pentazocine are very similar to morphine. Increasing the dose does not cause a corresponding increase in effect (27.5).

b) T Naloxone reverses the effects of morphine and other opioids including partial agonists such as pentazocine and nalorphine (27.5). Remember that naloxone itself is not totally devoid of unwanted effects and in some situations can be hazardous. See Questions 120, 178.

c) T Pentazocine has the ability to cause dysphoria which may be accompanied by nightmares and hallucinations (27.5).

d) T Pentazocine is a mixed agonist–antagonist or partial agonist (27.5). Receptor dualism is common amongst the opioids. This intriguing concept explains how some drugs may be agonists at one receptor type yet antagonists at another. The mu antagonist and kappa agonist drug nalbuphine is a good example.

e) T In binding studies pentazocine has a higher affinity for kappa (κ) receptors than for mu (μ) receptors. There is also behavioural evidence that pentazocine acts on sigma (σ) receptors (27.5). If the Greek alphabet is confusing a copy can be found in the Science Data Book (27.6).

28a) T Lignocaine is an aminoacyl derivative of acetanilide which possesses vasodilating activity. It is thus often mixed with adrenaline or another vasoconstrictor such as octapressin to prolong its duration of action (28.1).

b) T Lignocaine is metabolized in the liver by the microsomal mixed function oxidases by dealkylation to monoethylglycine xylidide and glycine xylidide, both of which are active metabolites with local anaesthetic properties. Xylidide is further metabolized before excretion in the urine (28.2).

c) T Lignocaine is one of many local anaesthetic agents that are amides. It is an aminoacyl amide (28.1). Esters are very little used today.

d) F The pKa of lignocaine at 25°C is 7.6 (28.3). The importance of the pKa value is to inform as to the pH value at which the agent is 50% ionized.

e) T Lignocaine is a weak base. It is, however, poorly soluble in water and thus is supplied as lignocaine hydrochloride solution which is acidic (28.4).

29 Oxytocic drugs have a wide variety of actions which do not always concern the uterus. It is foolish to assume that the routine use of oxytocic agents during caesarean section implies their lack of undesirable effects. The truth is very different.

The rapid i.v. injection of oxytocin causes:
a) hypotension
b) vasoconstriction
c) diuresis
d) hypertension
e) arrhythmias

30 Atropine is used therapeutically for many reasons. It reappears here as a reflection of its frequency of use in practice. Be aware of the actions of the drug when used in excess and in cases of acute poisoning. The completions in this question have a different emphasis to those met previously in Question 14.

The use of atropine is associated with:
a) malignant hyperpyrexia
b) skin rashes
c) confusion
d) mydriasis
e) neuromuscular blockade

References

29.1 Rang & Dale	p 551–553	
29.2 BNF	section 7.1.1	
30.1 Miller	p 950	
30.2 BNF	section 1.2	
30.3 Vickers, Morgan & Spencer	p 295–297	

29a) T When given intravenously the vasodilating effect of oxytocin will produce a transient fall in blood pressure (29.1).

b) F Oxytocic drugs have a vasodilating effect on the vasculature (29.1) which leads to a fall in arterial pressure.

c) F There is a weak vasopressin-like antidiuretic action which can result in water intoxication in some circumstances (29.1). This corresponds to the structural similarity of the molecule to vasopressin (ADH).

d) T In spite of the initial fall in systemic arterial pressure there may follow a sustained rise. Severe hypertension may be precipitated in the presence of pressor drugs (29.2). Changes in the tone of the pulmonary vasculature are common. Patients may complain of chest tightness and burning.

e) T Arrhythmias are cardiovascular side-effects of oxytocin (29.2). These may be supraventricular or, more rarely, ventricular in origin.

30a) F Although a raised body temperature may occur due to its physiological effects, atropine is not quoted as one of the trigger agents of malignant hyperpyrexia (30.1).

b) T Skin rashes occur, especially in poisoning, but are rare (30.2).

c) T Confusion and delirium may be seen with high doses. Atropine, being a tertiary amine, crosses the blood–brain barrier (see earlier). Quaternary ammonium compounds such as glycopyrronium bromide are less lipid soluble and less likely to cross the blood–brain barrier (30.2).

d) T Atropine is a standard mydriatic agent (when used topically). There is dilatation of the pupil with loss of accommodation and sensitivity to light (30.2). This effect may be prolonged.

e) F Atropine is a muscarinic antagonist. It has no effect at nicotinic receptors. Beware! Although atropine is commonly used in the reversal of competitive neuromuscular block, this is purely to prevent the unwanted muscarinic effects of anticholinesterases. It is not the only drug which can be used for this purpose (30.3).

31 There has already been a question on propranolol in this section but it is not unusual to find a recurring topic with a different emphasis or approach in the same examination. The change of approach may help, hinder, or confuse. Be cautious before changing the answer to a previous question.

Beta-blockers may cause:
a) hypotension
b) hypoglycaemia
c) reduced cardiac output
d) bronchospasm
e) skin rashes

32 Methaemoglobinaemia can appear as a topic in pharmacology or physiology. It can also appear in real life! Do not confuse drugs which cause methaemoglobinaemia with those used in its treatment.

The following may cause methaemoglobinaemia:
a) prilocaine
b) sodium nitrite
c) sodium nitroprusside
d) nitrous oxide
e) sulphonamides

References

31.1	Goodman & Gilman	p 229–241
31.2	BNF	section 2.4
31.3	Goodman & Gilman, 5th edn	p 552
32.1	Vickers, Morgan & Spencer	p 213–214
32.2	Goodman & Gilman	p 1630–1631
32.3	Vickers, Morgan & Spencer	p 349–351
32.4	Recent Advances 16	p 21
32.5	Atkinson, Rushman & Lee	p 395

31a) **T** Beta blockers cause a slowly developing reduction in blood pressure in patients with hypertension but not in normotensive patients. The mechanism of this effect is not fully understood (31.1).

  b) **F** Beta blockade masks the metabolic and autonomic symptoms of hypoglycaemia. In addition there may be a deterioration of glucose tolerance in diabetics. As a group, beta blockers are not totally contraindicated in diabetic patients (31.2).

  c) **T** Cardiac output and heart rate are decreased in beta blockade. These effects vary in magnitude with individual drugs, mainly due to variance in intrinsic sympathomimetic activity which is seen with different molecules. (31.1).

  d) **T** Bronchodilatation is an adrenergic $beta_2$ response. Beta blockers cause an increase in airway resistance and occasionally bronchospasm, especially in asthmatics (31.1).

  e) **T** Skin rashes may necessitate the withdrawal of treatment as they may reflect an allergic response to the drug (31.3).

32a) **T** This is a well recognized effect of prilocaine. Methaemoglobinaemia occurs with doses above 0.9 g in adults and results in cyanosis (32.1).

  b) **T** Sodium nitrite is used to oxidize haemoglobin to methaemoglobin in the treatment of cyanide poisoning (32.2).

  c) **T** Sodium nitroprusside may yield methaemoglobinaemia although this effect is not seen in small doses (32.3).

  d) **F** It is the higher oxides of nitrogen which cause methaemoglobinaemia (32.4). This is a classic red herring. Beware of the odd bell ringing if you are not entirely certain of the connection.

  e) **T** Sulphonamides are well known to cause methaemoglobinaemia (32.5). They may not immediately spring to mind in this regard but the statement is true.

33 The blood–brain barrier and placental barrier are both important when considering the sites of action and effects of drugs. It is essential to know how and why these barriers are different to other membranes and why their permeability to drugs differs.

The following cross the blood–brain barrier:
a) dopamine
b) suxamethonium
c) GABA
d) propranolol
e) edrophonium

34 The ideal induction agent is a dream. Take care to avoid confusion between the dream and the reality. The characteristics of an ideal induction agent nevertheless form a useful framework for both oral discussion and MCQ questions.

An ideal intravenous induction agent:
a) will be stable in solution
b) will be water soluble
c) will be lipid soluble
d) crosses the placenta
e) has a pKa of 11

References

33.1	Goodman & Gilman	p 466
33.2	Calvey & Williams	p 14–15
33.3	Rang & Dale	p 600–601
33.4	BNF	section 2.4
34.1	Aitkenhead & Smith	p 175–177
34.2	Vickers, Morgan & Spencer	p 15–18

33a) F Injected dopamine has no central effect because it does not cross the blood–brain barrier (33.1). It is precisely because of this that L-dopa is used as a treatment in Parkinson's disease. L-dopa is converted to dopamine after penetrating the blood–brain barrier.

b) F Suxamethonium is a quaternary ammonium compound. These are not able to cross the blood–brain barrier (33.2) because of their structure.

c) F GABA (gamma aminobutyric acid) itself fails to cross the blood–brain barrier, unlike its more lipid-soluble analogues. The *p*-chlorophenol derivative (baclofen) is one of these (33.3) and has been used in the treatment of spasticity due to its effect on muscle tone.

d) T The more lipid soluble beta blockers cross the blood-brain barrier easily and may cause sleep disturbance and dreams. Propranolol is an example (33.4) and the effect is featured in Question 1.

e) F Edrophonium is a quaternary ammonium compound. It is therefore highly ionized in the body and will not cross the blood–brain barrier (33.2).

34a) T Short-term stability in a solvent that can safely be injected is essential. Long-term stability in a simple solvent (water) would be the ideal (34.1).

b) T Water solubility is ideal and simple (34.1). It is generally the solubility (or rather the lack of it) in suitable solvents that has led to a great deal of trouble. A classic example is the former induction agent Althesin (alphaxolone and alphadolone) which was fated to be solubilized in Cremophor EL (polyoxylated castor oil) with the consequent problems of that vehicle.

c) T Lipid solubility is essential in order to enable the agent to cross the blood–brain barrier and reach its preferred site of action, the neurolipid (34.1). A corollary is that lipid soluble agents are difficult to formulate as a water-based solution. There is no such thing as a free lunch!

d) F Although this will almost certainly be a corollary of the lipid solubility it is not necessarily an ideal characteristic (34.1) and is undesirable.

e) F An ideal induction agent has a pKa close to plasma pH in order to achieve the compromise of water and lipid solubility which is necessary to achieve both aqueous solutions and penetration of neurolipid (34.2).

35 The following knowledge is of immense practical importance. It is also desirable to know the Vaughan Williams classification of antiarrhythmic drugs (35.1). This will be frequently encountered in Parts 2 and 3 of the FRCAnaes examination. The references have tables that can be memorized.

Which of the following have a place in treating VT:
a) disopyramide
b) digoxin
c) lignocaine
d) flecainide
e) verapamil

36 Do not confuse miosis and mydriasis. Miosis is pupillary constriction (36.1). Look again at Question 7 if you have any difficulty in recalling the definition of mydriasis.

Miosis is associated with:
a) alpha blockers
b) neostigmine
c) guanethidine
d) edrophonium
e) carbachol

References

35.1 BNF	section 2.3.2
35.2 Goodman & Gilman	p 818–820
35.3 BNF	section 2.3.1
36.1 BNF	section 11.6
36.2 Miller	p 488
36.3 Goodman & Gilman	p 137
36.4 BNF	section 11.6
36.5 Goodman & Gilman	p 126

35a) T Disopyramide is useful in the treatment of both supraventricular and ventricular tachycardias especially following acute myocardial infarction (35.1).

b) F Ventricular refractory period is reduced by digoxin; ventricular excitability is increased. Digoxin is valuable in the treatment of supraventricular tachycardias (35.2).

c) T Lignocaine remains the first line treatment of ventricular arrhythmias. The newer derivatives like flecainide are also useful (35.3).

d) T Flecainide is indicated in the treatment of ventricular tachycardia and can also be used for junctional re-entry tachycardias. It lies in the same class (class I) as lignocaine in the Vaughan Williams classification (35.1).

e) F Verapamil is the recommended treatment for supraventricular tachycardias (35.1). Beware clinically of the negative inotropic effect of verapamil.

36a) T Pupillary constriction occurs dependent on the level of pre-existing parasympathetic tone (36.2).

b) T When applied topically, constriction of the sphincter pupillae muscle produces miosis. The ciliary muscle also contracts so blocking the accommodation reflex with resultant focusing to near vision only (36.3).

c) T Topical application of guanethidine initially produces mydriasis with increased aqueous outflow which is later followed by miosis with reduced aqueous outflow (36.4). Note the earlier comment in Question 7 concerning the uncertainty over the mydriasis. No such debate occurs with regard to the miotic action.

d) T As edrophonium is an anticholinesterase, miosis will occur although there is no preparation available for topical ocular use (36.3).

e) T Carbachol is a choline ester. Carbachol intraocular solution can be instilled into the anterior chamber during ocular surgery to produce miosis (36.5).

37 The overlap between pharmacology and physiology can be marked; the same questions may appear under both headings. This can also happen in both pharmacology and physiology vivas, which may be good or bad luck! The catecholamines provide an example.

The infusion of noradrenaline results in:
a) a rise in systolic pressure
b) a fall in diastolic pressure
c) a fall in mean arterial pressure
d) a fall in heart rate
e) a rise in pulmonary vascular resistance

38 Most questions concern the normal use of drugs in patients. There is, however, no reason why questions should not be asked about drugs in overdose. These may be illustrative of their applied pharmacology.

Aspirin overdose results in:
a) hypothermia
b) hypoglycaemia
c) oedema
d) acidosis
e) coma

References
37.1 Ganong   p 337–338
37.2 Goodman & Gilman   p 194

38.1 Calvey & Williams   p 341–343
38.2 Goodman & Gilman   p 651

37a) T The vasoconstriction that noradrenaline produces via alpha$_1$ receptors increases total peripheral resistance. There is only a small decrease in cardiac output due to reflex bradycardia. Generally systolic pressure rises (37.1).

b) F Diastolic pressure rises along with systolic pressure. Conversely, with infusion of adrenaline the diastolic pressure falls (37.1).

c) F If both systolic and diastolic pressure rise then the mean pressure must rise (37.1). This should be obvious from the calculation of mean arterial pressure.

d) T Bradycardia occurs as a result of the baroreceptor reflex which overrides any direct cardioacceleratory effect of noradrenaline (37.1).

e) T Noradrenaline and adrenaline are both capable of increasing pulmonary artery pressure (37.2).

38a) F Whilst therapeutic doses of aspirin will lower body temperature in febrile patients, toxic doses will produce hyperthermia due to increased oxygen consumption and metabolic rate associated with abnormal cellular respiration (38.1).

b) F Hypoglycaemia may occur with therapeutic doses of all salicylates due to increased tissue utilization of glucose. In toxic doses hyperglycaemia may occur because of increased activity of the adrenal medulla and cortex (38.1). Hypoglycaemia may result from toxic doses in young children (38.2). This completion is possibly best marked as a don't know.

c) F Both dehydration and pulmonary oedema may occur in salicylate poisoning but peripheral oedema is not recorded (38.2). The assumption made in this completion (reasonably) is that peripheral oedema is being referred to rather than pulmonary oedema.

d) T Acid-base changes with high-dose aspirin treatment and overdose are complex. In toxic doses the respiratory centre is depressed producing a respiratory acidosis. Metabolic acidosis will also occur due to dissociation of salicylate and derangement of carbohydrate metabolism (38.1).

e) T As the pattern of aspirin poisoning progresses, central stimulation changes to increasing depression of conscious level, stupor, and coma (38.2). There is thus a confusing biphasic pattern in overdosage.

39 Antagonists of calcium transport have come to the fore recently. In the main this is due to the increasing popularity of the group in the treatment of hypertension. The interaction of calcium antagonists and inhalational anaesthetic agents is a subject of concern and research.

Antagonists of calcium transport include:
a) verapamil
b) dantrolene
c) sodium nitroprusside
d) baclofen
e) digoxin

40 It would not be representative of the real examination if statistics were absent, for at least one question on this subject is guaranteed. Very few people enjoy learning about statistical analysis and it is one of the least popular revision topics, but the subject is absolutely inescapable in the examination and to ignore it in revision is suicidal. There are some very good, basic texts available and one of these is 'Statistics at square one' by Swinscow, see Bibliography.

Standard deviation:
a) is the square root of variance
b) is a measure of population scatter
c) only applies to normally distributed data
d) is an estimate of skewness
e) can be calculated from the range and the mean

References		
39.1 BNF		section 2.6.2
39.2 Vickers, Morgan & Spencer		p 265–266
39.3 Calvey & Williams		p 432–433
39.4 Rang & Dale		p 704
39.5 Rang & Dale		p 325–327
40.1 Swinscow		p 7–15

39a) T Verapamil is a calcium channel blocker. It interferes with the inward displacement of calcium ions through the slow channels of active cell membranes. Verapamil is principally used for the treatment of angina, hypertension, and supraventricular arrhythmias (39.1).

b) T Dantrolene uncouples excitation–contraction coupling by interfering with the release of ionic calcium from the sarcoplasmic reticulum (39.2).

c) T Sodium nitroprusside may inhibit the influx, binding, and translocation of calcium ions in vascular smooth muscle. It may also affect excitation-contraction coupling in skeletal muscle (39.3).

d) F Baclofen is a chlorophenol derivative of GABA which has a selective action at $GABA_B$ receptors (39.4). Do you know enough about the subclassification of GABA receptors?

e) F The increase in myocardial contraction is produced by an increase in the size of the intracellular calcium transient, possibly due to a greater release of calcium from intracellular stores which ensures greater availability (39.5).

40a) T The square root of the variance is the standard deviation (40.1).

b) T Standard deviation is a useful measure of the scatter of observations of a population (40.1).

c) F The population should approximately fall into a normal (or Gaussian) distribution (40.1).

d) F Skewness is a layman's term and is not valid in statistics. Standard deviation is a measure of the range of observations from a mean (40.1).

e) F Standard deviation is calculated from the differences from the mean and is a measure of the range of observations (40.1).

41 The second batch of 40 questions concerns physiology. The first two questions relate to the crucial topic of respiratory physiology, a thorough knowledge of which should be second nature to any serious Part 2 FRCAnaes candidate. The physiology section may have a welcome clinical relevance as demonstrated below.

The application of 10 cm of PEEP:
a) will cause death within a few minutes
b) reduces cardiac output
c) will cause a rise in intracranial pressure
d) causes a fall in Pa_{O_2}
e) causes closure of alveoli

42 The various shifts in the oxygen haemoglobin dissociation curve must be understood in detail. When the direction of the shifts is incorrectly recalled minus marks become a certainty. If in doubt try drawing the curve and marking the axes. An aide memoire for the factors involved and the direction of shift that each one causes will undoubtedly be an advantage. When practising drawing the curve check the labelling of the axes; mistakes are common.

The oxygen haemoglobin dissociation curve:
a) will shift to the left in hypothermia
b) has a P_{50} of 27 mmHg
c) has a sigmoid shape
d) will shift to the right if 2, 3-DPG is reduced
e) is affected by carbon monoxide

References	
41.1 Atkinson, Rushman & Lee	p 293
41.2 Nunn	p 417–419
41.3 Miller	p 2186–2189
42.1 Ganong	p 617–619
42.2 Aitkenhead & Smith	p 39
42.3 Nunn	p 264
42.4 Churchill Davidson	p 131
42.5 Nunn	p 266

41 The essential item missing from this question is '10 cm of what?' One is forced to assume that 10 cm H_2O PEEP (positive end expiratory pressure) is implied. This has deliberately not been turned into an idealized question by quantifying the units.

a) **F** This is untrue in any but the most parlous clinical states but pressures above 16 cm H_2O may cause an increase in interstitial and alveolar water (41.1). In extremis, death might be an event within a few minutes of the introduction of PEEP but it is safe to exclude that reasoning. The response here should clearly be 'false'.

b) **T** The fall in cardiac output, which is usually not seen in moderate levels of PEEP, is secondary to decreased venous return to the heart which reduces preload. Other factors of importance include increased right ventricular afterload (due to higher pulmonary capillary resistance), decreased left ventricular compliance, and reduced myocardial contractility. The respective importance of each of these is debatable (41.2).

c) **T** Intrathoracic venous pressure and intracranial pressure will both rise in parallel with the application of PEEP (41.1). The latter effect should be borne in mind when the cerebral circulation is embarrassed, for example in global head injury with cerebral oedema. In the clinical situation a value judgement needs to be made as to whether a gain in oxygenation is worth the price of the deleterious cardiovascular effects of PEEP.

d) **F** The purpose of PEEP is to open closed alveoli (alveolar recruitment—not usually seen with levels of PEEP below 10 cm H_2O), to increase FRC, and improve oxygenation. However, in hypovolaemic patients 10 cm H_2O PEEP may produce such a fall in cardiac output that Pa_{O_2} may decrease (n.b. a fall in Pa_{O_2} is strictly speaking pathology not physiology!) (41.3).

e) **F** PEEP increases the diameter of patent alveoli and recruits previously collapsed ones. In this way FRC is actually increased (41.3).

42a) T It is essential to know which factors change the oxyhaemoglobin dissociation curve and in which direction (42.1). In general, items that decrease or fall move the curve to the left, and thus hypothermia, a <u>fall</u> in temperature, does so.

b) **T** The P_{50} is 27 mmHg or 3.5 kPa. This represents that oxygen tension at which haemoglobin is 50% saturated. In normal subjects the value varies between 3.5 and 3.9 kPa (42.2) (42.3).

c) **T** The characteristic sigmoid-shaped curve is due to the quaternary structure of haemoglobin which results in an increasing affinity for the binding of subsequent oxygen molecules to haem after the first binding has taken place (42.1).

d) **F** Certain organic phosphates within the erythrocyte were found experimentally to have a profound effect on P_{50}. 2, 3-Diphosphoglycerate (2, 3-DPG) is the most important of these. One molecule of 2, 3-DPG binds preferentially to the beta chains of one tetramer of deoxyhaemoglobin causing a functional change which reduces oxygen affinity. A decrease in 2, 3-DPG will thus cause a shift of the curve to the <u>left</u> (42.1, 42.5).

e) **T** Carbon monoxide causes the formation of carboxyhaemoglobin and subsequent to this there is a shift to the left of the dissociation curve of the remaining oxyhaemoglobin (42.4).

43 The scope of respiratory physiology is extensive. Of all the areas in which you are likely to be examined this is the most common. Consider this question logically. Take each completion together with the stem as one statement and consider it in isolation. Do not allow yourself to be distracted by another completion but rather answer each singly. There are no 'tricks'.

At the end of a deep expiration:
a) basal alveoli will be gas free
b) all airways will contain alveolar gas
c) the lungs will be at FRC
d) pulmonary compliance is reduced
e) mixed venous oxygen content will fall

44 Detail on the formation and drainage of cerebrospinal fluid is not difficult to obtain as it is featured in many standard texts. Some anatomical knowledge of the choroid plexus is advantageous. Revise the composition of CSF as well as its circulatory paths.

Cerebrospinal fluid:
a) is produced by the choroid plexus
b) is absorbed by the arachnoid villi
b) contains very little glucose
d) provides the only source of nutrition to the brain
e) contains high levels of protein

References	
43.1 West	p 159–160
43.2 Ganong	p 602–604
44.1 Ganong	p 563–564
44.2 Dunnill & Colvin	p 85

43a) F By definition the end of deep expiration means that the lungs are at residual volume (RV). Although at this volume many of the airways in lower lung regions are closed, gas may be trapped in the alveoli when airways close and it is thus very unlikely that they will be gas free (43.1).

b) T Anatomical dead space is approximately 150 ml for an average adult. In reaching residual volume from a position of normal exhalation the loss of expiratory reserve volume (ERV) is 1 litre. All dead space gas has thus been cleared and therefore only alveolar gas can remain in the airways (43.2).

c) F Functional residual capacity (FRC) is the volume of gas left in the lungs after normal expiration as opposed to maximal expiration, when the lungs will be at residual volume. See above (43.2).

d) T The reduction in compliance is thought to be due to a change in alveolar configuration (43.1) although the precise cause is not yet fully understood.

e) F Closed airways will result in an unfavourable ventilation/perfusion ratio and arterial hypoxia. However, a single deep expiration is insufficient to transmit any such changes through the vascular system to the mixed venous content (43.1).

44a) T About 50–75% of CSF is formed in the choroid plexus. The remainder is formed around the cerebral vessels and along the ventricular walls. In the human the turnover of CSF is approximately four times per 24 h (44.1).

b) T CSF flows through the foramina of Magendie and Luschka and is absorbed through the arachnoid villi thence passing into the cerebral venous sinuses (44.1).

c) F CSF glucose amounts to 2.2–4.5 mmol/l, or approximately 1.1 mmol/l less than blood glucose (44.2).

d) F The main function of CSF is to support the brain and protect against physical shocks. Nutrition is supplied by the blood (44.1). Some workers have suggested that CSF may have a minor nutritional role. This is uncertain. CSF is certainly not the only source of nutrient to the brain.

e) F The total amount of protein in CSF is between 150 and 400 mg/l. This is considerably less than in the plasma (44.2). CSF protein levels may reach higher values in pathological conditions.

45 It is always wise to be wary of statements in medicine which incorporate 'always'. Be certain of the facts before committing yourself. A line of discrimination needs to be drawn here between passive and active hyperventilation both of which share some, but not all, features of the process.

Passive hyperventilation always causes:
a) a fall in Pco_2
b) a rise in Po_2
c) an increase in free calcium ions
d) a fall in pH
e) a fall in bicarbonate

46 The control of cardiac output is complex yet logical. In anaesthetic practice it is manipulated every day and a high level of knowledge will be expected. The definition of moderate exercise is essential to answer the first completion.

Cardiac output:
a) increases in moderate exercise
b) may be measured by the Fick method
c) increases with a rise in Pco_2
d) increases if stroke volume rises
e) falls when IPPV is started

References
45.1 Atkinson, Rushman & Lee   p 78–79
45.2 West   p 132

46.1 Ganong   p 526–532
46.2 Current Anaesthesia and Critical Care
         (1989) 1.1   p 4

45 Passive hyperventilation (as in mechanical ventilation) does not involve effort on the part of the subject. Active hyperventilation increases the metabolism of muscles resulting in raised carbon dioxide production (45.1) but there will usually be a fall in P_{CO_2} due to the respiratory effect of hyperventilation.

a) T Intermittent positive pressure ventilation (IPPV) conventionally employed during general anaesthesia usually reduces Pa_{CO_2} which may fall to 3 kPa or less (45.1). This may be adjusted in modern practice by the more frequent use of capnography.

b) F Passive hyperventilation with unaltered FI_{O_2} will not elevate P_{O_2}. There may be tissue hypoxia from the reduction in cardiac output; there is also a shift of the oxyhaemoglobin dissociation curve to the left (45.1) due to respiratory alkalosis.

c) F A fall in ionized calcium will be seen with a slight increase in total plasma calcium concentration (45.1).

d) F The pH rises. This is a direct effect of the respiratory alkalosis (45.1).

e) F Although renal compensation will occur for a respiratory alkalosis by excretion of bicarbonate this process may take 24 h to occur. Hyperventilation thus does not always cause a fall in bicarbonate (45.2).

46a) T Heart rate increases and stroke volume shows a modest increase in normal subjects; therefore cardiac output increases (46.1). Moderate exercise does not involve anaerobic metabolism as distinct from severe exercise where an oxygen debt is inevitable.

b) T The Fick principle states that the amount of a substance taken up by an organ per unit of time is equal to the arterial level of the substance minus the venous level, in other words the A–V difference. This principle is used for indicator techniques of measurement of cardiac output (46.1) whether by thermal or dye dilution.

c) T A rise in P_{CO_2} acts as a vasodilator and also causes sympathetic stimulation. Although the former may reduce preload and thus cardiac output, the latter is a potent stimulus to increased cardiac output (46.1) and has the greater effect.

d) T This statement is true if one assumes peripheral resistance and heart rate remain constant (46.1). The effect most frequently observed on commencing IPPV is a fall in arterial pressure resulting from the lessening of preload which is itself due to raised intrathoracic pressure. This effect may have a lesser magnitude when high-frequency ventilation techniques are used because of the minimal effect on intrathoracic pressure (and thus venous return) that low tidal volumes produce.

e) T Reduced cardiac output is the result of the rise in mean intrathoracic pressure which produces a fall in preload (46.2).

47 The key to answering this question correctly is to be able to define 'moderate' haemorrhagic shock. For those who remain uncertain Ganong (47.1) refers. It is advised most strongly that definitions such as this (and those of moderate and severe exercise) are memorized.

In moderate haemorrhagic shock:
a) there is an increase in physiological dead space
b) there is increased pulmonary shunt
c) arteriovenous oxygen content difference increases
d) central venous pressure falls
e) plasma renin levels will rise

48 Neurophysiology is featured in detail in the examination. Particular topics of interest are the various pathways of the nervous system. In this question some answers may be deduced from elementary knowledge of the functions of the cerebellum. Some clinical knowledge is necessary too.

If the cerebellum is non-functional:
a) voluntary movement is jerky
b) intention tremor is present
c) constant tremor is present
d) the finger–nose test is positive
e) basal ganglia cannot function normally

References	
47.1 Ganong	p 588–590
47.2 Nunn	p 377
47.3 Nunn	p 173
47.4 Shoemaker	p 150–153
48.1 Ganong	p 201–206
48.2 Macleod	p 275
48.3 Ganong	p 198–201

47   Moderate haemorrhagic shock is defined as the loss of 5–15 ml/kg
body-weight (47.1). Remember this definition!

a) T Physiological dead space is increased in both haemorrhagic
hypotension and hypotension induced by ganglionic blockade.
The textbook explanation is that pulmonary hypotension causes
failure of perfusion of the uppermost parts of the lung fields.
Note, however, that this has not been confirmed experimentally
(47.2).

b) F There is no evidence of increased pulmonary shunting during
haemorrhagic hypotension (47.2). This situation is sometimes
cited as evidence of pulmonary shunting being in direct proportion to cardiac output (47.3). This would imply in shock that
falling cardiac output defrays any potential increase in shunting.

c) T In haemorrhagic shock there are increases in heart rate, peripheral vascular resistance, arteriovenous oxygen difference, and
also oxygen extraction (47.4).

d) T The central venous pressure (CVP) falls in shock, as does the arterial
pressure, cardiac output, total blood volume, central blood volume,
stroke volume, left ventricular stroke work, oxygen delivery, and
oxygen uptake (47.4).

e) T There is increased renin and aldosterone secretion (47.1) which
will both tend to act, teleologically speaking, as protective
mechanisms. _takes 30 min to work_

48a) T Intention tremor with jerky purposeful movements is characteristic of cerebellar dysfunction. All movements are ataxic (ataxia
is defined as incoordination due to errors in the rate, force, and
direction of movement) (48.1).

b) T Intention tremor is typically present. Cerebellar lesions cause no
signs until purposeful movement is initiated (48.1). By way of
contrast, resting tremor is observed in Parkinsonian states.

c) F Humans with lesions of the cerebellum show no signs whilst at
rest (48.1).

d) T Dysmetria (or past pointing) occurs when the attempt to touch an
object with a finger results in overshooting to one side or another
(48.1). The test is positive when the result is abnormal (48.2).

e) F The basal ganglia comprise the caudate nucleus, putamen, and
globus pallidus. It appears that the major role of the basal ganglia
is to convert abstract thought into actual movement. The cerebellum is not part of the efferent pathway from the basal ganglia
(48.3) which should be able to function normally without the
cerebellum.

49 Candidates are often required to draw diagrams to illustrate the various lung volumes and capacities. This question is based along those lines. It may help to draw a diagram before attempting this one. Make sure you can put numerical values on each volume and capacity.

The components of vital capacity include:
a) functional residual capacity
b) tidal volume
c) residual volume
d) inspiratory reserve volume
e) expiratory reserve volume

50 Every MCQ paper is likely to contain material relating to renal physiology. Special heed should be paid to the measurement of glomerular filtration rate and renal plasma flow and the differences between them. A dedicated revision text on renal physiology represents money well spent.

In the normal kidney:
a) GFR may be estimated by PAH clearance
b) renal plasma flow is around 500 ml/min
c) the tubular maximum for glucose is 375 mg/min
d) sodium reabsorption is always passive
e) urinary pH lies between 3 and 10

References	
49.1 Nunn	p 39
50.1 Ganong	p 656
50.2 Ganong	p 653–654
50.3 Ganong	p 661
50.4 Ganong	p 660
50.5 Ganong	p 671

49a) F The components of vital capacity are best seen on a spirometer trace of static lung volumes (49.1). Vital capacity comprises expiratory reserve volume, tidal volume, and inspiratory reserve volume. Part of the functional residual capacity (residual volume) lies below the volume of the lungs at maximal expiration and FRC is not therefore a component of vital capacity (49.1).

b) T Tidal volume is a component of vital capacity (49.1).

c) F Residual volume (RV) lies between zero lung volume and the lung volume at maximal expiration (which is the lower limit of vital capacity). Learn the diagram of lung volumes and capacities. It is essential to differentiate between volumes and capacities (49.1).

d) T Inspiratory reserve volume (IRV) is part of vital capacity (49.1).

e) T Expiratory reserve volume (ERV) is that extra volume of gas which may be expired after the end of normal tidal expiration. ERV is a component of FRC (49.1).

50a) F Inulin clearance is used to measure glomerular filtration rate (GFR), as it is freely filtered and neither secreted nor reabsorbed (50.1). Para-aminohippuric acid (PAH) is used to measure renal plasma flow (50.2).

b) F Renal plasma flow is 625 ml/min (50.3).

c) T The tubular maximum for glucose (Tm_G) is about 375 mg/min in men and 300 mg/min in women (50.4). Tubular maxima for glucose are not identical between tubules and this splay of values is a popular examination theme. *desc LOH*

d) F Sodium ions are actively transported out of all parts of the renal tubule except the thin portions of the loop of Henle (50.4).

e) T Urine pH in normal subjects is 4.5–8.0 (50.5). The normal range of 4.5–8.0 does lie between 3 and 10, but 3 and 10 is not the normal range. This is a good example of a question that is very easy to misread and lose a mark when you do actually know the correct answer. *Sneaky*

51 This first question on metabolism concerns antidiuretic hormone (ADH). The involvement of this hormone with the pituitary gland may provide an opening gambit in vivas. Sometimes ADH and vasopressin are used in the same question. They may be considered synonymous.

Antidiuretic hormone:
a) has a plasma half-life of 24 h
b) increases cyclic AMP in the collecting tubule
c) increases water permeability in the proximal tubule
d) is produced in the anterior pituitary
e) can cause systemic vasoconstriction

52 With regard to the adrenal gland a frequent cause of lost marks is confusion between those hormones manufactured in the adrenal medulla and cortex respectively. Think clearly before attempting to answer.

Hormones produced in the adrenal cortex include:
a) adrenaline
b) angiotensin II
c) aldosterone
d) fludrocortisone
e) deoxycorticosterone

References	
51.1 Lote	p 91–93
51.2 Ganong	p 224–225
52.1 Ganong	p 339–359
52.2 Ganong	p 426–427
52.3 Rang & Dale	p 522

51a) F As the primary hormone responsible for the maintenance of plasma osmolality it is necessary that ADH is both rapidly secreted in response to dehydration and rapidly removed from plasma. ADH is excreted 10% in the urine and the remainder is metabolized. The plasma half life is 10–15 min (51.1).

b) T In the collecting tubule the hormone receptor complex for ADH activates adenyl cyclase which catalyses the formation of cyclic 3,5-AMP (adenosine monophosphate) from ATP. The ADH receptors are thought to be on the peritubular side rather than the luminal side of the tubular cells (51.1).

c) F ADH regulates plasma osmolality by changing urine volume, that is, by altering the permeability of the collecting ducts to water. A distinction is made between V_1 receptors mediating vasoconstriction and V_2 receptors mediating the antidiuretic effects of the hormone. V_2 receptors are present in the ascending loop of Henle and collecting ducts, not in the proximal convoluted tubule (51.2).

d) F ADH is synthesized in the supraoptic nucleus of the hypothalamus and transported via the hypothalamo-hypophyseal nerve tract to the neurohypophysis (posterior pituitary). ADH is released from the posterior pituitary (51.1).

e) T ADH is a potent vasoconstrictor although the effect is mediated through different receptors (V_1) to those involved in the antidiuretic action (V_2) (51.2).

52 The hormones of the adrenal cortex are derivatives of cholesterol which are converted to steroids (52.1).

a) F Catecholamines such as adrenaline are produced by the adrenal medulla and not by the cortex. This completion always catches somebody out! (52.1).

b) F Angiotensin II is produced by conversion from angiotensin I by angiotensin converting enzyme (ACE). The enzyme is located in endothelial cells, particularly within the lungs but is found in many other tissues. ACE may also be referred to as kininase 2 (52.2).

c) T The adrenal cortex produces the mineralocorticoids aldosterone and deoxycorticosterone, the glucocorticoids cortisol and corticosterone, and the androgens dehydroepiandrosterone and androstenedione (52.1).

d) F Fludrocortisone is a synthetic steroid with potent mineralocorticoid activity and little glucocorticoid activity. It is used as replacement therapy in Addisonian states to ameliorate the loss of aldosterone (52.3).

e) T Deoxycorticosterone is one of the hormones secreted by the adrenal cortex (52.1).

53 The sympathetic nervous system is intimately connected with adenylate cyclase. A knowledge of applied pharmacology will prove useful here. The detailed structure of the adrenoceptor is relevant and it is necessary to be aware of the different effects of alpha and beta ligands (both subtypes $_1$ and $_2$) on the same.

Adenylate cyclase:
a) converts ATP to cyclic AMP
b) is an enzyme
c) is the adrenergic receptor
d) is inhibited by theophylline
e) is activated by phenylephrine

54 A classic question on respiratory physiology, if there is such an animal, might be exemplified by the one below. Despite its elementary nature the question is very searching and therefore efficient at sorting wheat from chaff.

In normal quiet breathing:
a) the bases of the lung expand more than the apices
b) the external intercostal muscles raise the ribs
c) the abdominal muscles aid expiration
d) the strap muscles are inactive
e) closing volume approaches FRC

References

53.1	Ganong	p 37–39
53.2	Ganong	p 88–94
53.3	Rang & Dale	p 741–742
53.4	Rang & Dale	p 184
53.5	Nimmo & Smith	p 147
53.6	Goodman & Gilman	p 207
53.7	AHFS	p 631
54.1	Nunn	p 142–143
54.2	Ganong	p 604
54.3	Ganong	p 602–603
54.4	Nunn	p 62–63

53a) T True, although it might be more proper to refer to adenylate cyclase as a catalyst for the conversion of ATP to cyclic AMP (cAMP) within the cell. Nonetheless the conversion is enzymatic (53.1).

b) T Adenylate cyclase is the enzyme responsible for the formation of cAMP from ATP (53.1).

c) F Although the effects of both $beta_1$ and $beta_2$ receptor stimulation are brought about by activation of adenylate cyclase with a consequent increase in intracellular cyclic AMP, the actual adrenergic receptor is complex, comprising stimulatory and inhibitory receptors and stimulatory and inhibitory 'G' proteins. In summary $beta_1$ and $beta_2$ receptors involve G stimulatory proteins while $alpha_2$ receptors involve G inhibitory proteins. $Alpha_1$ receptors, on the other hand, produce their effect by activating $phospholipase_3$ (53.1) (53.2).

d) F Methylxanthines (especially theophylline) inhibit the enzyme phosphodiesterase, which is responsible for the metabolism of cAMP (53.3).

e) F Phenylephrine acts mainly via $alpha_1$ receptors (53.4). $Alpha_1$ receptors modify calcium channel control (53.5). However, in large doses phenylephrine has weak beta effects (53.6). A further source states: 'Phenylephrine acts predominantly by a direct effect on alpha adrenergic receptors. In therapeutic doses the drug has no substantial effect on beta adrenergic receptors. It is believed that alpha adrenergic effects result from the inhibition of the production of cAMP' (53.7).

54a) T In normal tidal respiration there is a ratio of 1.5 : 1 in favour of basal ventilation although postural effects should also be considered. At inspiratory flow rates greater than 1.5 l/s, however, uniform ventilation is seen (54.1).

b) T Movement of the diaphragm accounts for 75% of the change in intrathoracic volume during quiet inspiration. The other important inspiratory muscles are the external intercostal muscles, which run obliquely downwards and forwards from rib to rib. These muscles raise the lower ribs in quiet respiration (54.2).

c) F Expiration during quiet breathing is passive in the sense that no muscles which decrease intrathoracic volume contract (54.3).

d) T The scalene and sternocleidomastoid muscles in the neck are accessory inspiratory muscles which help to elevate the thoracic cage during deep laboured ventilation (54.2). They are usually demonstrated par excellence on any urological list when half the patients listed for TURP appear to be respiratory cripples.

e) F The convergence of closing volume and FRC is age dependent. In adults below the age of 60 years closing volume should be less than FRC. During quiet breathing closure will not occur (54.4). Note that closing capacity is equal to closing volume plus residual volume (54.4).

55 A frequent source of confusion is the differentiation of the respective roles of carotid body and carotid sinus. The carotid body has a chemo-receptor role whereas the carotid sinus has a mechanoreceptor role. The relationships of each are complex.

The carotid body responds to:
a) a fall in pH
b) increased P_{CO_2}
c) a fall in blood pressure
d) doxapram
e) increased traffic in the buffer nerves

56 Haematological subjects may appear in the context of the examination. Red cell morphology is one of these and the physiology of clotting is certainly another. Think especially carefully before attempting the completion on half life in this question.

Red blood cells:
a) have nuclei
b) have an increased volume in the peripheral circulation
c) can utilize energy from anaerobic pathways
d) have a half life of 30 days
e) have a higher respiratory quotient than parietal cells

References

55.1	Guyton	p 201
55.2	Guyton	p 446–450
55.3	AHFS	p 1182
55.4	Ganong	p 556–557
55.5	Ganong	p 625–626
56.1	Ganong	p 490
56.2	West	p 74–76
56.3	Wintrobe	p 103
56.4	Oxford Textbook of Medicine	section 19. 65–66
56.5	Ganong	p 457–458

55a) T The carotid body contains chemoreceptors which respond to local changes in hydrogen ion concentration (55.1). If hydrogen ions increase in concentration (a <u>fall</u> in pH) then arterial pressure rises by an effect which is mediated through the vasomotor centre.

b) T Both central and peripheral chemoreceptors are sensitive to the partial pressure of carbon dioxide in their perfusant (55.2).

c) T A fall in blood pressure below a critical level will cause stimulation of the chemoreceptors. This occurs because of a reduction in blood flow through the carotid bodies which restricts oxygen availability at tissue level. A rise in CO_2 and a drop in local pH will contribute to this response (55.1).

d) T The action of doxapram is primarily one of direct stimulation of the medullary respiratory centres. There is, however, reflex activation of both carotid and aortic chemoreceptors (55.3).

e) F The term 'buffer nerves' describes the carotid sinus nerves and vagal fibres from the aortic arch. These are baroreceptor fibres (55.4). Afferents from the carotid body ascend to the medulla via the carotid sinus and glossopharyngeal nerves. Fibres from the aortic bodies ascend in the vagi (55.5).

56a) F In the circulation of mammals red cells have no nuclei, these having been lost previously in the bone marrow (56.1).

b) T The uptake of CO_2 by red cells increases their osmolarity and consequently water enters the cells thus increasing their net volume (56.2). The corollary of this is that shrinkage occurs during passage through the lung as CO_2 is lost.

c) T Erythrocytes metabolize glucose. Under normal circumstances 90% of glucose entering the red cell is metabolized by the anaerobic glycolytic (Embden–Meyerhof) pathway. The remaining 10% is metabolized by the aerobic pentose phosphate pathway (otherwise known as the hexose monophosphate shunt or phosphogluconate pathway) (56.3).

d) F The life <u>span</u> of red cells is on average 120 days and can be assessed in many ways. Chromium[51] is used to label red cells to determine sites of destruction. The half-life of the label ^{51}Cr in labelled red cells is 25–36 days. Take care (56.4).

e) T Parietal cells are distinguished by having a negative respiratory quotient (56.5).

57 The lung is an organ of great importance to anaesthetists. Apart from the obvious roles of the lung, non-respiratory aspects of pulmonary function should be included in any revision plan. The completions that follow this stem are a mix of mechanics and metabolism.

In the lung:
a) hysteresis can be prevented by the application of PEEP
b) the law of Laplace applies
c) the pleural pressure gradient falls during inflation
d) catecholamines are metabolized
e) total compliance is equal to the sum of the compliances of the lung and thorax added together

58 Surfactant features regularly in major journals as our understanding of it improves—another good reason for keeping abreast of the periodicals.

Pulmonary surfactant:
a) is decreased by increased F_{IO_2}
b) is a lipoprotein
c) is produced by type II pneumocytes
d) is decreased in premature babies
e) is decreased in a segment if blood flow is reduced

References
57.1 Nunn	p 28–31
57.2 Ganong	p ~~606–607~~ 328
57.3 Current Anaesthesia and Critical Care (1989) 1.1	p 4
57.4 West	p 47–48
57.5 West	p 101–102
58.1 Atkinson, Rushman & Lee	p 62
58.2 Ganong	p 606
58.3 Guyton	p 404–405
58.4 Nunn	p 15–20
58.5 West	p 92–93

57a) F Hysteresis occurs when the pressure/volume curve for static points during <u>inflation</u> differs from that during <u>deflation</u>. This phenomenon is present to a greater or lesser extent in all elastic bodies (57.1). PEEP does not alter the elastic properties of the lungs although it does cause an increase in FRC.

b) F Alveoli collapse in accordance with Laplace's law unless surface tension is reduced by surfactant (57.2).   Pg S28

c) T In spontaneous ventilation expansion of the rib cage and descent of diaphragm alter the subatmospheric intrapleural pressure from −5 cm H_2O to −10 cm H_2O (57.3).

d) T Noradrenaline is metabolized in the lung (54.4) which has a role in the metabolism of catecholamines generally. Compare Question 80.

e) F Total compliance of the lung and the chest wall is the sum of the <u>reciprocals</u> of the lung and chest wall compliances measured separately (57.5). Don't get caught out by the wording.

58a) T Surfactant may be reduced in oxygen toxicity and after prolonged artificial ventilation especially when large tidal volumes need to be employed (58.1).

b) T The lipoprotein surfactant is composed of the phospholipid dipalmitoylphosphatidylcholine (DPCC) and two major proteins, one of molecular weight 32 000 Daltons and the other of molecular weight 10 000 Daltons (58.2).

c) T Surfactant is secreted by special cells, type II granular pneumocytes (58.3). There are a number of special cell types at alveolar and bronchial level (types I, II and III). Nunn (58.4) refers.

d) T A few newborn babies, especially premature babies, do not secrete adequate quantities of surfactant which makes lung expansion difficult due to very low compliance (58.3).

e) T If the blood flow to a region of lung is abolished the surfactant there may be depleted. A good example is seen in pulmonary embolism (58.5).

$$P = \frac{2T}{r}$$

P = transmural pressure
T = Tension
r = radius

59 The cytochrome system is intimately concerned with metabolism at a cellular level. It might be thought that this is an obscure subject but the examiners may not agree. There is ample detail available in textbooks to study, for example Nunn (59.2).

Cytochrome P$_{450}$
a) is found in lysosomes
b) is bright red in colour
c) is an anaerobic dehydrogenase
d) is found in the carotid body
e) is only found in reticulocytes

60 For those of us who are not specialists in gastrointestinal medicine there is only one method of defence against a question like this. Learn the factors affecting gastric emptying, parrot-fashion.

Gastric emptying into the duodenum:
a) is increased by fat in the stomach
b) is inhibited by acid in the duodenum
c) is enhanced by cholecystokinin
d) is delayed by gastrin
e) is related to the volume of gastric contents

References
59.1 Ganong   p 14
59.2 Nunn   p 242
59.3 Harper   p 107
59.4 Nunn   p 84

60.1 Ganong   p 459–461
60.2 Ganong   p 449–454
60.3 Guyton   p 702–703

59a) F Lysosomes are organelles within a cell that contain a variety of enzymes which would cause destruction of most cellular components if the enzymes were not separated from the rest of the cell. Lysosomes function as a form of digestive system for the cell and contain ribonuclease, deoxyribonuclease, phosphatase, glycosidases, arylsulfatases, collagenase, and cathepsins. There is no cytochrome P_{450} (59.1). Cytochrome P_{450} is present in cell microsomes (smooth endoplasmic reticulum) of various organs such as liver, kidneys, lung, intestinal mucosa, and skin (59.2).

b) F Cytochromes, which are porphyrin-containing proteins, can be classified by their absorption spectra. For example, cytochrome P_{450} after carbon monoxide absorption has a maximal absorption of light at 450 nm (59.2). In absorption spectrophotometry 430 nm is violet and 470 nm is blue. The absorption of this light leads to a bright red appearance. All cytochromes in their normal state appear sludgy red–brown to the eye.

c) T Cytochromes are iron-containing haemoproteins which are classified as anaerobic dehydrogenases (59.3).

d) F Cytochrome P_{450} is not present in the carotid body. Cytochrome a_3 is, however, present therein. This cytochrome is a special type which is 50% reduced at a high level of P_{O_2} (12 kPa). It is thought that this cytochrome may actually be the P_{O_2} sensor (59.4).

e) F Cytochrome P_{450} is ubiquitous (59.1) and can be found in several organs.

60a) T The presence of fat in the stomach inhibits gastric emptying (60.1). This effect has been used prophylactically by revellers over the years to slow the rate of absorption of alcohol.

b) T Fats, carbohydrates, and acid in the duodenum inhibit gastric acid and pepsin secretion and gastric motility. This is probably mediated via gastric inhibitory peptide and other hormones that inhibit gastric emptying (60.1).

c) F The main functions of cholecystokinin are to produce contraction of the gallbladder and encourage the secretion of pancreatic juice but it also inhibits emptying and may enhance motility of the small intestine and colon (60.2).

d) F The main physiological actions of gastrin are to stimulate secretion of gastric acid and pepsin and promote growth of gastric mucosa. Gastrin may also stimulate gastric motility (60.3).

e) T The rate at which the stomach empties is determined by signals both from the stomach and from the duodenum. The stomach signals are mainly twofold: nervous—caused by distension of the stomach by food; and hormonal—gastrin is released from the antral mucosa in response to the presence of certain types of food in the stomach (60.3).

61 The electrophysiology of the electrocardiogram (ECG) will often be met. The duration of the various phases is purely a test of memory but more understanding is necessary to relate the events of the cardiac cycle to the electrical signals.

The QRS complex of the ECG:
a) has a duration of less than 0.2 s
b) represents the period of ventricular contraction
c) varies in amplitude with respiration
d) has the same voltage all over the chest wall
e) is temporally related to the A wave of the JVP

62 With regard to questions on biochemistry the best advice one can give is 'Do not panic'. Some of the completions below can be worked out by applying basic principles.

Plasma ionized calcium concentration:
a) is increased by hyperventilation
b) is decreased by parathormone
c) falls with decreased pH
d) is unaffected by calcitonin
e) is increased by 1,25-dihydroxycholecalciferol

References
61.1 Guyton   p 118–123
61.2 Ganong   p 507–510
61.3 Goldschlager & Goldman   p 42–43

62.1 Atkinson, Rushman & Lee   p 78–79
62.2 Ganong   p 367–369
62.3 Miller   p 1450–1452

61a) T The normal QRS duration is 0.08–0.10 s (61.1). This phase represents the period of ventricular depolarization.

b) F The QRS complex occurs at the start of phase 2 of the cardiac cycle (the phase of isovolumetric contraction). The QRS complex is complete by the start of phase 3 (ventricular ejection). The T wave (ventricular repolarization) also occurs during ventricular contraction (61.2). Learn the cardiac cycle in detail and note the point at which the aortic and ventricular pressure curves cross.

c) T In normal quiet breathing there is no change in amplitude of the ECG. However, on deep inspiration the position of the heart becomes more vertical in relation to the chest so that QRS complex morphology changes, resulting in a change in amplitude (61.3).

d) F The amplitude of deflection changes across the V or chest leads in line with the voltage (61.1).

e) T The A wave of the JVP (jugular venous pressure) is due to atrial systole which coincides with the QRS complex at the start of phase 2 of the cardiac cycle (61.2).

62a) F In hyperventilation there is a fall in plasma-ionized calcium but a slight increase in total plasma calcium (62.1).

b) F Parathormone (PTH) is a hormone essential to life. After parathyroidectomy there is a steady decline in plasma calcium levels (62.2).

c) T Plasma ionized calcium concentration is influenced by pH directly. It is thus important that samples for analysis are taken under anaerobic conditions (62.3). This may not always be the case in practice.

d) F Calcitonin lowers the plasma calcium and phosphate levels (62.2).

e) T The hormone 1, 25-dihydroxycholecalciferol acts on the intestine and bone to increase ionic plasma calcium and phosphate (62.2).

$Ca^{2+} \downarrow \quad pH \downarrow \quad acidosis$

Apparent Total $Ca \uparrow \bar{c}$ venous stasis

∴ hyperproteinaemia

63 There has been a wealth of research into the physiology of pain transmission, and some great advances have been made to deepen our perception of nociception since the original concept of the pain 'gate' was described.

The transmission of pain:
a) occurs via the spinothalamic tracts
b) arises from nociceptors
c) involves peptidergic pathways in the CNS
d) involves synaptic transfer within the substantia gelatinosa
e) is inhibited by descending pathways

64 The liver has a central role in metabolism. Its functions include various syntheses and biochemical conversions as well as regulatory functions (64.1). Drawing on clinical experience of liver failure may prove useful.

Functions of the liver include:
a) manufacture of plasma proteins
b) secretion of bile
c) gluconeogenesis
d) manufacture of antibodies
e) acetylation

References
63.1 Wall & Melzack   p 12
63.2 Wall & Melzack   p 22–45
63.3 Scurr, Feldman & Soni   p 346–347
63.4 Scurr, Feldman & Soni   p 349–352
63.5 Wall & Melzack   p 52–53

64.1 Ganong   p 465–467
64.2 Guyton   p 751–752
64.3 Guyton   p 773
64.4 Roitt   p 20–24
64.5 Calvey & Williams   p 24

63a) T The spinothalamic tract is generally regarded as the most important pathway for signalling painful stimuli in humans (63.1). This is elementary.

b) T Although some authorities make a distinction between pain and nociception (63.2), it is generally thought that nerve endings which respond to painful stimuli are nociceptors (63.3).

c) T All the endogenous neurotransmitters for pain are peptides. Apart from the obvious families of endorphins, enkephalins and dynorphins, other examples include substance P and vasointestinal peptide (VIP) (63.4). An expanding area of interest is the primary nociceptive transmitter—neuropeptide K—otherwise known as neurokinin A.

d) T The dorsal horns are divided on a histological basis. Laminae II and III of Rexed make up the substantia gelatinosa (63.3). There are three types of afferent fibre of which the small unmyelinated C fibres are concerned primarily with pain and temperature (63.5).

e) T Descending inhibition is a major factor and has a considerable degree of complexity (63.4).

64a) T The manufacture of plasma proteins is one of the major roles of the liver (64.1). Reduced levels of plasma proteins frequently accompany liver failure.

b) T For an easy mark this is hard to beat (64.1). If you got this wrong give up now.

c) T Gluconeogenesis is the formation of carbohydrates from proteins and fats (64.2). In the liver this function is concerned with maintaining normal blood glucose (64.3).

d) F Plasma cells are the site of production of antibodies (64.4). This completion is a distractor.

e) T Drug acetylation may occur in several tissues. Examples include gastrointestinal mucosa, kidney, and liver (64.5).

65 The response to major injury presents a very similar metabolic picture to the response to surgery. The parallels should be immediately obvious. Postoperative fluid requirements are based on a knowledge of electrolyte changes. Consideration of these may be a useful manœuvre before attempting to answer.

In the first 24 hours after major injury:
a) sodium is retained
b) potassium is lost
c) metabolic rate is increased
d) urinary nitrogen levels will fall
e) plasma osmolality is unchanged

66 This question is very broad based and will test the knowledge of any candidate over a wide area. A similar interrogative could be used with respect to potassium.

With respect to sodium:
a) the daily requirement in man is 5 g
b) it is actively transported in the proximal convoluted tubule
c) it is the main intracellular anion
d) it is lost in the urine obligatorily
e) it is a major component of bile

References
65.1 Atkinson, Rushman & Lee   p 749
65.2 Miller   p 2297

66.1 Atkinson, Rushman & Lee   p 795
66.2 Guyton   p 317
66.3 Guyton   p 276–278
66.4 Lote   p 110–111
66.5 Guyton   p 721–722

65a) T After major injury sodium excretion is impaired. This phase may last from 4 to 6 days and is independent of sodium intake (65.1).

b) T In sharp contrast to the situation with respect to sodium, potassium excretion is increased. This phase reaches a maximum in 24 h and terminates within 48 h (65.1).

c) T In the initial post-trauma period glucagon, catecholamines and glucocorticoids are secreted leading to protein catabolism. Unlike the catabolism of uncomplicated starvation, insulin control of the hyperglycaemia is difficult (65.2).

d) F There is an increase in urinary nitrogen excretion which may exceed 16 g/24 h (65.2). Catabolism is thus marked which is unsurprising.

e) F ADH secretion is stimulated and this can lead to a fall in serum osmolality. Note, however, that aldosterone secretion is also increased which may reduce the effect (65.2).

[handwritten: 1L N/Saline = 150mmol per day]

66a) F The normal sodium requirement for an average adult is 100 mmol/ 24 h, in other words 2.3 g/24 h (66.1). Remember that requirement will increase by 50 mmol for each degree Celsius rise in temperature.

b) T There is an active transport system for sodium in the proximal convoluted tubule. Sodium entry into the cell is down a large electrical and chemical gradient and passive movement occurs by this mechanism (66.2).

c) F Intracellular sodium concentration is 14 mmol/l in comparison to a concentration of more than 130 mmol/l in extracellular fluid. The main intracellular anion is potassium (66.3).

d) T There is a certain mandatory loss of ions and water: the 'volume obligatoire'. Urinary sodium loss is normally 20 mmol/24 h less than intake and can fall to a very low level when necessary. The obligatory sodium loss by all routes is about 30 mmol/24 h. In situations of restricted intake sodium excretion in the urine can fall to very low levels, down to a few mmol/24 h (66.4).

e) T Sodium is the largest ionic component of bile at 130–145 mmol/l (66.5). Gall bladder bile has a lower sodium content than hepatic bile.

[handwritten notes:]

Urinary Nitrogen

N   35mg/kg /24hr   2.5g / 24hr

Trauma (Catabolism)   16 g / 24hr

Starvation (catabolism)   10 g / 24hr

67 Most of the uncertainty surrounding the secretions of the pituitary gland results from confusion as to which are properly pituitary in origin and which are secreted by the hypothalamus.

The pituitary gland secretes:
a) prolactin
b) corticotrophin releasing factor
c) FSH
d) long acting thyroid stimulator
e) vasopressin

68 If the metabolic response to starvation has not been included in your revision then it would be wiser in the actual examination itself to ignore this type of question. Starvation presents a complex metabolic picture not commonly encountered outside an intensive care unit.

In starvation:
a) urinary nitrogen falls
b) ketogenesis occurs
c) glucagon levels are raised
d) cerebral glucose uptake is increased
e) there is metabolic acidosis

References	
67.1 Ganong	p 373–374
67.2 Guyton	p 838–839
68.1 Ganong	p 279–280
68.2 Shoemaker	p 1128
68.3 Ganong	p 280–282
68.4 Ganong	p 327–328
68.5 Ganong	p 572
68.6 Tweedle	p 231

67a) T The pituitary gland secretes prolactin from the anterior lobe (67.1).

b) F Corticotrophin releasing factor, in common with several other releasing factors, is produced by the hypothalamus (67.1).

c) T FSH stands for follicle stimulating hormone. This is another of the anterior lobe pituitary hormones (67.1).

d) F LATS is long acting thyroid stimulating factor. It is an antibody formed by the plasma cells and is thought to bind to receptors in the thyroid gland. The result is activation of cyclic AMP and general cellular stimulation (67.2).

e) T Vasopressin (antidiuretic hormone) is secreted by the posterior lobe of the pituitary gland (67.1). *V₁ vasocon. DAG / V₂ ADH cAMP*

68a) F In complete starvation, where there is no protein sparing effect of carbohydrates, urea nitrogen excretion averages 10 g/24 h as proteins are catabolized for energy (68.1). Normal urinary nitrogen excretion is 35 mg/kg 24 h^{-1} in the adult male and somewhat less in the female (68.2).

b) T Leucine, isoleucine, phenylalanine, and tyrosine are all ketogenic amino acids (68.3). *PILT*

c) T Glucagon secretion increases during starvation and reaches a peak on the third day of the fast. At this time the gluconeogenesis is maximal (68.4). Glucagon itself has a ketogenic action (see above).

d) F Glucose is the major source of energy for the brain under normal conditions resulting in a respiratory quotient for the tissue of 0.95–0.99. In prolonged starvation the brain can use other sources (68.5). It is interesting to note that substances other than glucose are metabolized during convulsions—a situation of acute, severe metabolic demand.

e) T Metabolic acidosis can occur in starvation. This is probably due to the increase in ketones (68.6).

69 Although the phase of sleep known as 'rapid eye movement' (REM) may seem an obscure subject it remains a favourite in the examination. REM sleep is covered in some detail in standard physiology textbooks.

In REM sleep:
a) skeletal muscle tone is increased
b) cerebral blood flow rises
c) dreaming occurs
d) erections are common
e) there is high frequency activity on the EEG

70 When attempting to answer a question such as this it may prove useful to draw on knowledge of applied pharmacology in order to elucidate the physiological mechanisms involved.

Bowel peristalsis:
a) is stimulated by muscarinic agonists
b) will be abolished in high spinal cord transection
c) is inhibited by eating
d) is inhibited by coeliac plexus stimulation
e) is unaffected by hormones

References	
69.1 Guyton	p 659–660
69.2 Atkinson, Rushman & Lee	p 43
70.1 Goodman & Gilman	p 125
70.2 Oxford Textbook of Medicine	section 21.107
70.3 Guyton	p 703–705

69a) F The muscle tone throughout the body is exceedingly depressed during REM sleep. This is due to inhibition of spinal projections from the reticular formation of the brain stem (69.1).

b) T There is an increase in cerebral blood flow during REM sleep (69.2).

c) T Dreams occur during REM sleep and these may be exceedingly vivid in nature (69.2).

d) T Tumescence of the penis occurs resulting in erection (69.2).

e) T Beta waves occur during REM sleep. These are waves with a frequency of 14–50 cycles/s. Slow wave activity occurs during Non-REM sleep (NREM) (69.1).

70a) T Muscarinic agonists demonstrate the effects of acetylcholine on the gastrointestinal tract. These include an increase in peristalsis (70.1).

b) F Following spinal cord injury peristalsis ceases, either immediately if the abdomen has been injured, or else within 24 h as a result of spinal shock. These patients often show gastric dilatation and paralytic ileus for a few days (70.2).

c) F Peristalsis is increased by the distension in the bowel wall which occurs after eating (70.3).

d) T Coeliac plexus stimulation leads to sympathetic activation which inhibits peristalsis (70.3).

e) F Several hormones influence the motility of the bowel. Secretin, for example, causes a reduction in motility (70.3).

71 The main problem of describing the regulation of calcium is ensuring that the effects of the regulatory factors are recalled correctly. This is particularly important when considering the action of parathormone on the renal tubules.

Parathormone:
a) is a polypeptide
b) increases phosphate excretion
c) increases calcium reabsorption from bone
d) requires vitamin A as a coenzyme
e) responds to variations in serum calcium

72 When it is a simple matter of factual recall, you either know it or you don't. Do not confuse internal intercostals with external. This is a common error.

The following are muscles of expiration:
a) diaphragm
b) internal intercostals
c) external intercostals
d) rectus abdominus
e) scalenus anterior

References

71.1 Ganong   p 367–371

72.1 Ganong   p 604

71a) T Human parathormone is a polypeptide of molecular weight 9500 Daltons. It contains 84 amino acid residues (71.1).

b) T Phosphate excretion is enhanced by a direct phosphaturic action. The reabsorption of phosphate in the proximal tubule is decreased. Note that calcium reabsorption in the <u>distal</u> tubule is increased (71.1). Be careful in this convoluted area.

c) T The action of parathormone in bone involves the activation of cyclic AMP. The permeability of osteoblasts to calcium in bone fluid is increased. The osteoblasts then pump calcium into the extracellular fluid (ECF) (71.1).

d) F Vitamin A is principally involved in visual acuity. Vitamin D is needed for the absorption of calcium and phosphates (71.1).

e) T The circulating level of ionized calcium acts directly on the parathyroid gland to regulate the secretion of parathormone (71.1).

72a) F The diaphragm is a muscle of inspiration (72.1). It is possible to work this out from the anatomy of the muscle. Contraction of the diaphragm will increase thoracic volume.

b) T The internal intercostals pull the rib cage downwards as they contract and aid expiration (72.1).

c) F The external intercostals have the opposite effect to the internals (72.1) and aid inspiration. There is thus a mnemonic to be found here: **EXT**ernal intercostals for **INSP**iration and **INT**ernal intercostals for **EXP**iration.

d) T The muscles of the abdominal wall aid expiration by increasing intra-abdominal pressure (72.1). They are important in forced expiration and coughing.

e) F The scalene muscles are accessory muscles of inspiration and have no role in expiration (72.1).

73 The physiological response to acute haemorrhage is featured here. More information is given in the stem than is usual: a value for the loss, for example. Consider the responses you would make if the stem read **'acute haemorrhage will cause'**.

In a healthy adult a sudden blood loss of 500 ml will cause:
a) tachycardia
b) increased peripheral vascular resistance
c) increased ADH secretion
d) sudden collapse
e) fall in diastolic pressure

74 The fact that detailed knowledge of cardiovascular physiology is required for this examination cannot be stressed highly enough. Pay particular attention to the circulation through special regions, which is often featured in textbooks as a dedicated topic. The coronary circulation is one of these but others include the blood flow through brain and kidney.

Coronary artery blood flow:
a) has diastolic pressure as its main determinant
b) is unaffected by changes in arterial pressure
c) is under humoral control
d) is reduced in severe tachycardia
e) at rest is about 2 l/min

References	
73.1 Atkinson, Rushman & Lee	p 743
73.2 Ganong	p 226–227
74.1 Guyton	p 237–240
74.2 Ganong	p 573–576

73a) T Loss of up to 15% (750 ml) of the blood volume results in a normal blood pressure with tachycardia and postural hypotension (73.1).

b) T A loss of up to 1000 ml of blood is usually well compensated by splanchnic and cutaneous vasoconstriction (73.1) together with tachycardia.

c) T Although ADH is primarily a hormone for osmotic control, ECF volume also affects ADH (vasopressin) secretion. Haemorrhage is a potent stimulus to ADH secretion (73.2).

d) F The loss of 10% (500 ml) of the blood volume is well tolerated with little effect on arterial pressure and cerebral perfusion (73.1).

e) F As mentioned above, the blood pressure will usually not change with losses of 10% or less of the blood volume (73.1).

74a) T Diastolic pressure is a more important determinant of coronary artery blood flow for the left rather than right ventricle (74.1). Endomural wall tension is prohibitively high in systole; it is during diastole that coronary blood flow occurs. This is an important physiological point with relevance to disease states.

b) F Arterial pressure changes will influence coronary artery blood flow both by changing the driving pressure and the ventricular intraluminal pressure (74.1).

c) F Blood flow through the coronary system is regulated almost entirely by a vascular response to the local needs of the cardiac musculature for nutrition (74.1).

d) T Blood flow to the left ventricle occurs mostly during diastole. Since diastole is shorter when the heart rate is rapid, left ventricular coronary blood flow is reduced during tachycardia (74.2).

e) F A flow of 2 l/min is approaching half the total cardiac output! The average coronary blood flow is approximately 225 ml/min or 0.7–0.8 ml/g of heart muscle min^{-1} or 4–5% total cardiac output (74.1).

75 Hypomagnesaemia may be met in clinical practice. Magnesium is principally an intracellular electrolyte with an effect on neuromuscular irritability. Magnesium deficiency is characterized by disorientation and somnolence amongst other symptoms.

Hypomagnesaemia:
a) is characterized by muscle weakness
b) may cause cardiac arrhythmias
c) may cause convulsions
d) is a complication of aminoglycoside therapy
e) causes a prolonged Q–T interval

76 Blood flow through special regions can appear in both parts of the examination. Cerebral circulation is just one example from this category. While the stem is similar to Question 74 the completions are very different, reflecting the various control mechanisms of each system.

Cerebral blood flow:
a) exhibits large regional variations
b) is greater than coronary artery blood flow
c) is highly susceptible to changes in local Po_2
d) is subject to autoregulation
e) is affected by local release of kinins

References
75.1 Atkinson, Rushman & Lee   p 83
75.2 Miller   p 276
75.3 Rang & Dale   p 163
75.4 Atkinson, Rushman & Lee   p 282
75.5 Rowlands   section 2, p 263
75.6 Braunwald   p 217

76.1 Guyton   p 679–681
76.2 Ganong   p 551–552

75a) T Clinical signs associated with low magnesium include tremors, twitching, tetany, muscular weakness, confusion, and hallucinations (75.1).

b) T Clinical effects of hypomagnesaemia include cardiac arrhythmias. These are principally ventricular tachyarrhythmias (75.2).

c) T The sequelae of hypomagnesaemia include neuromuscular irritability such as tremors, twitching, asterixis, and seizures (75.2).

d) F This question attempts to create an association that does not exist. Among agents that inhibit calcium entry and potentiate neuromuscular blockade are both magnesium ions and aminoglycoside antibiotics. It can be easy to extrapolate such an erroneous association under examination conditions (75.3) (75.4).

e) F There are at least 12 causes of a prolonged Q–T interval including: hypocalcaemia, hypothermia, intracranial haemorrhage, hypothyroidism, acute cor-pulmonale, and long Q–T syndrome! (75.5). ECG effects of hypomagnesaemia cannot be demonstrated (75.6).

76a) T Regional variations in cerebral blood flow change rapidly with different activities (76.1). This reflects the relevant neuronal involvement on a geographical basis within the brain.

b) T The average cerebral blood flow is 0.5–0.55 ml/g min^{-1}, or 750 ml/min for the whole brain. This represents 15% of the total cardiac output (76.1). Coronary artery blood flow is 0.7–0.8 ml/g min^{-1} or approximately 225 ml/min.

c) T Carbon dioxide increases cerebral blood flow by raising hydrogen ion concentration. The fall in pH causes vasodilatation in direct proportion (76.1).

d) T Cerebral blood flow is autoregulated extremely well between the pressure limits of 60 and 140 mmHg (76.1). The plot of perfusion against pressure is a curve that you should be prepared to reproduce on paper.

e) T Kinins cause vasodilatation. A kinin-like peptide has been implicated as a possible cause of migraine (76.2).

77 A large number of factors including drugs may affect blood glucose concentration. This question might easily appear in the pharmacology section with different completions.

Blood glucose concentration is increased by:
a) cortisol
b) noradrenaline
c) growth hormone
d) thyroxine
e) lipolysis

78 The morphological changes in muscle during shortening are difficult to visualize. This is definitely an occasion where a drawing will provide some assistance. A very useful and clear diagram may be found in 'Gray's Anatomy' (78.1) which is not a text one would normally associate with revision for the Part 2 FRCAnaes.

During muscle shortening changes occur in the length of the:
a) A band
b) H zone
c) Z line
d) I band
e) muscle spindles

References

77.1	Guyton	p 846–847
77.2	Ganong	p 324
77.3	Guyton	p 823
77.4	Ganong	p 302–304
77.5	Oxford Textbook of Medicine	section 8.10
78.1	Gray's Anatomy	p 547–553
78.2	Ganong	p 116–121

77a) T Both the increased rate of gluconeogenesis and the moderate reduction in the rate of glucose utilization by the cells induced by cortisol will cause the blood glucose concentration to rise (77.1).

b) T Noradrenaline inhibits insulin secretion (as does sympathetic stimulation of the pancreas) which results in a rise in blood glucose. Note that hepatic factors are also important (77.2).

c) T Initially, on injection of growth hormone into an animal, cellular uptake of glucose is enhanced and blood glucose concentration falls. The effect lasts approximately 30 min and then a more prolonged reverse effect occurs. Beware! (77.3).

d) F Thyroxine has a 'calorigenic' action causing an increase in metabolic rate. There is no increase in blood glucose. However, thyroid hormones increase the rate of absorption of carbohydrate from the gastrointestinal tract, and in hyperthyroidism the blood glucose level rises rapidly after a carbohydrate meal to then fall again rapidly. Answer at your peril (77.4). The answer quoted is the authors' choice.

e) F Lipolysis occurs during food deprivation or insulin deficiency and may therefore occur when the blood glucose is elevated. Lipolysis is defined as the breakdown of fats to non-esterified fatty acids for use as an energy substrate. There is no accompanying rise in blood glucose (77.5).

78a) F The A band represents the myosin filaments of the sarcomere. It is not a change in actual filament length but rather a sliding of actin filaments on myosin filaments that is responsible for shortening of the sarcomere (78.1).

b) T The H zone is the area lying between the ends of the actin filaments in which are the myosin filaments. As the sarcomere shortens, the ends of the actin filaments approximate so reducing the H zone (78.1).

c) F The Z line is the junction between sarcomeres and does not change during contraction (78.1).

d) T The I band describes the area between the ends of the myosin filaments within which the Z line is placed centrally. As the sarcomere shortens, the ends of the myosin filaments approach the Z line so reducing the I band (78.1).

e) T Muscle spindles consist of 2–10 muscle fibres enclosed in a connective tissue capsule. They contract and shorten when the gamma efferents are stimulated (78.2).

79 It is possible to deduce some answers to this question from first principles. In the first instance the application of simple logic should give a clue to the first completion. The Valsalva manœuvre and its physiological effects deserve singling out as an exceedingly frequent topic in this examination. The effects of a change in posture from recumbent to standing may be an accompanying subject.

Peripheral resistance is increased in:
a) haemorrhage
b) changing from supine to standing
c) exercise
d) Valsalva manœuvre
e) high ambient temperature

80 The importance of the lung has been emphasized earlier. The non-respiratory roles of the lung have long been favoured by examiners. A list of non-respiratory pulmonary roles would be a useful revision aid.

The non-respiratory functions of the lung include:
a) metabolism of dopamine
b) metabolism of adrenaline
c) metabolism of serotonin
d) production of prostaglandin E_2
e) conversion of angiotensin I

References
79.1 Shoemaker   p 156
79.2 Ganong   p 583–584
79.3 Ganong   p 585–587
79.4 Ganong   p 558–559
79.5 Ganong   p 234–235

80.1 Nunn   p 284–293

79a) T Generalized vasoconstriction is a rapid compensatory mechanism which acts to increase peripheral resistance (79.1). It is logical that there should be a vasoconstrictor response to bleeding to protect the organism.

b) T Total peripheral resistance increases by 25% on standing (79.2). Remember this well.

c) F There is a fall in total peripheral resistance due to the vasodilatation which occurs in exercising muscles in response to metabolic demand (79.3).

d) T There is a rise in peripheral resistance to maintain the blood pressure as venous return falls within the thorax and preload becomes reduced. It is the ejection into a constricted vascular bed at the end of the Valsalva manœuvre which causes the short-lived hypertension and subsequent (reflex) bradycardia (79.4).

e) F Cutaneous vasodilatation will occur in an environment of high temperature. While this will aid heat loss and cooling, a reduction in peripheral resistance will be seen as a consequence (79.5).

80a) F Dopamine is largely unaffected by passage through the lung in contrast to 5-hydroxytryptamine and noradrenaline which are both extracted (80.1).

b) F Adrenaline is largely unaffected by passage through the lung in contrast to 5-HT and noradrenaline (80.1).

c) T Remember serotonin *is* 5-hydroxytryptamine. The lung is a very efficient extractor of 5-HT from the circulation. As much as 98% can be removed in a single pass. The mechanism is direct uptake into capillary endothelium followed by metabolism by monoamine oxidase; analogous to the fate of noradrenaline (80.2).

d) F The precursor of the prostaglandin family (prostaglandin G_2) is formed in the lung (80.1) but prostaglandin PGE_2 is formed by cyclo-oxygenase in macrophages.

e) T Angiotensin I undergoes biotransformation to angiotensin II in the lung (80.1). Angiotensin converting enzyme (ACE) is present in large amounts on the vascular surface of pulmonary endothelial cells.

81 Ketamine is seldom used today as a routine but kept for special situations. The pharmacology of the drug is markedly different from other induction agents which may make it easier to remember. Ketamine is indicated in the management of severe trauma at the site of accidents. It is part of most flying squads' armamentarium.

Ketamine may cause:
a) an increase in heart rate
b) postural hypotension
c) alpha blockade
d) rigidity
e) delirium

82 In contrast to ketamine, Hartmann's solution (sodium lactate intravenous infusion compound) is used daily in every hospital. The contents of the solution are written on the outside of each bag. Read it.

Hartmann's solution:
a) contains potassium ions
b) is iso-osmolar with extracellular fluid
c) has a pH of 7
d) is miscible with insulin
e) contains no phosphate

References
81.1 Vickers, Morgan & Spencer   p 64–65
81.2 Atkinson, Rushman & Lee   p 249
81.3 Calvey & Williams   p 176–178

82.1 Dunnill & Colvin   p 156
82.2 BNF   appendix 6

81a) **T** A rise in the heart rate of approximately 15 beats/min occurs after the intravenous administration of ketamine. Arterial pressure increases by some 25% and cardiac output is either unchanged or increased (81.1). Ketamine also increases myocardial workload.

b) **F** Arterial pressure is generally raised. Ketamine has been recommended for use when blood pressure needs to be maintained (81.2). In general, however, myocardial oxygen consumption increases and myocardial work is increased.

c) **T** Ketamine produces vasodilatation in tissues predominantly innervated by alpha adrenoceptors. Vasoconstriction occurs in tissues innervated by beta adrenoceptors. The sympathetic blockade is probably not at receptor level; as yet the true site of blockade is unknown (81.1).

d) **T** Hypertonus and spontaneous muscle movements may occur and jaw tone may be increased (81.3). The increase in muscle tone can be a practical problem in situations where ketamine is employed as the sole anaesthetic agent.

e) **T** Hallucinations, vivid dreams and emergence delirium may continue for up to 24 h after administration (81.3). This is said to be less of a problem in the very old and very young. Commonly benzodiazepine premedication is used to minimize these effects although the resultant success is variable.

82a) **T** Hartmann's solution (Ringer lactate) contains 5 mmol potassium/l (82.1). Hartmann's solution is frequently used in anaesthesia because its composition so closely resembles that of extracellular fluid.

b) **T** The osmolality of Hartmann's solution is 280 mosmol/l (82.1). This can be calculated from the ionic components and their concentrations.

c) **F** The pH of the solution is 6.5 (82.1).

d) **T** Most types of insulin may be mixed together with Hartmann's solution without incompatibility (82.2).

e) **T** Hartmann's solution does not contain any phosphate. However, magnesium and calcium are both present (82.1).

83 Sometimes a stem may say 'The following statements are true' and the completions that follow may cover five different subjects. In this case the subject in question concerns analgesic drugs in the broadest sense.

The following statements are true:
a) cannabinoids are analgesics
b) NSAI drugs inhibit cyclo-oxygenase
c) aspirin may be given intravenously
d) beta endorphin is a powerful analgesic
e) naltrexone has analgesic effects

84 Diazoxide was originally developed as an oral antihypertensive drug but proved to be unacceptably toxic. It remained available for intravenous use in hypertensive emergencies but sodium nitroprusside has almost completely replaced it. Diazoxide is still found in examination papers. Compare Question 6.

Diazoxide:
a) is related to the thiazides
b) is an antihypertensive agent
c) relaxes uterine muscle
d) produces hypoglycaemia
e) is a diuretic

References
83.1 Dundee, Clarke & McCaughey   p 425
83.2 Rang & Dale   p 284–285
83.3 BJA (1985) 57   p 255
83.4 Anaesthesia Review 3   p 56
83.5 Goodman & Gilman   p 515

84.1 Goodman & Gilman   p 804–805

83a) T Cannabinoids are analgesics themselves and also potentiate other analgesic agents (83.1). It is the better known effects of euphoria and sedation that make their recreational use popular.

b) T All the non-steroidal anti-inflammatory agents (NSAIDs) inhibit arachidonate cyclo-oxygenase. This inhibition can occur by different mechanisms. 1. An irreversible time-dependent inactivation of the enzyme (e.g. aspirin). 2. A rapid reversible competitive inhibition (e.g. propionic acid NSAIDs). 3. A rapid reversible non-competitive inhibition (e.g. paracetamol) (83.2).

c) F Aspirin is acetylsalicylic acid which is not available for intravenous (i.v.) use. There is a water soluble salt of acetylsalicylic acid—lysine salicylic acid—which is both water soluble and suitable for i.v. use. This drug has been compared favourably with i.v. morphine for postoperative pain relief (83.3).

d) T Beta endorphin is a powerful analgesic agent. An increased concentration of beta endorphin in CSF produces analgesia after being released by electrical stimulation of the periaqueductal grey matter (83.4).

e) F Naltrexone is a derivative of naloxone with a much longer half life and is a relatively pure antagonist. At high doses there are some agonist effects but they have little clinical significance (83.5).

84a) T Diazoxide is a benzothiadiazine derivative as are the thiazide diuretics. Diazoxide unusually shows sodium retaining effects. The molecule lacks the sulphonamido group of the thiazides (84.1).

b) T Arterial smooth muscle relaxes due to hyperpolarization of the muscle cells by the action of diazoxide on ATP-sensitive K^+ channels. In vivo the effect is exclusively arteriolar with a negligible effect on the capacitance vessels (84.1), in contrast to sodium nitroprusside.

c) T Diazoxide is a relaxant of uterine smooth muscle and if used to treat hypertension during labour may result in arrest of the labour (84.1).

d) F On the contrary. Hyperglycaemia results from the inhibition of the secretion of insulin from the pancreatic beta cells. There is no change in the cellular response to insulin (84.1).

e) F Water and sodium retention are common problems of treatment. They result from reflex activation of the sympathetic nervous system. Although belonging to the same class of drugs as the thiazide diuretics, diazoxide does not cause a diuresis because it lacks a sulphonamido group (84.1), hence the sodium retaining effect.

85 Every anaesthetist would like to claim that he or she never has the need of an analeptic. Nonetheless most pharmacy departments have continually to replenish stocks of doxapram. The claim of 'I never need such a drug' will not persuade a computer of widespread pharmacological knowledge and in a viva will probably result in some very searching questions. If you use it—know it.

Doxapram:
a) acts on the thalamus
b) increases tidal volume
c) raises arterial pressure
d) has a high therapeutic ratio
e) reduces cardiac output

86 Every effort is made to create questions that are well constructed but not every question is perfect. Be very careful answering questions which have 'may, never, or always' in the stem. In the case of 'may' in the following question the method of crossing a membrane will not always be one that is usually associated with drugs but one that may nonetheless occur.

Drugs may cross membranes by:
a) diffusion
b) pinocytosis
c) lipolysis
d) active uptake
e) secretion

References		
85.1 Data Sheet Compendium	p 1226	
85.2 Vickers, Morgan & Spencer	p 225–227	
86.1 Vickers, Morgan & Spencer	p 15–18	
86.2 Harper	p 149	
86.3 Goodman & Gilman	p 18	

85a) T Although doxapram stimulates respiration by affecting peripheral chemoreceptors and possibly also the respiratory centre, all levels of the CNS are stimulated (85.1).

b) T Doxapram causes an increase in tidal volume with rather less of an increase in respiratory rate (85.1).

c) T A small increase is seen in both blood pressure and heart rate mediated via the vasomotor centre and sympathetic nervous system. There is also a rise in cardiac output (85.2).

d) T The respiratory stimulating effects can be achieved with doses 40–60 times less than those needed to cause convulsions (85.2). Compared with the other analeptic agents it must be said that doxapram has a relatively high therapeutic ratio. The therapeutic ratio of the drug in absolute terms is not high.

e) F Rapid administration of doxapram can cause an increase in cardiac output (85.2).

86a) T Diffusion is the movement of a substance along a concentration gradient to the lower concentration. Diffusion can occur in the lipid phase of membranes (lipid diffusion) or through the pores in membranes (aqueous diffusion) depending on the relative solubility of the drug in the different media (86.1).

b) T In pinocytosis and phagocytosis drugs of large molecular weight, or drug aggregates, can be transported by being engulfed as small droplets and carried across the cell membrane (86.1).

c) F Lipolysis is the breakdown of fats by hydrolysis to fatty acids which are released into the circulation as free fatty acids (86.2). This completion is a red herring.

d) T Active uptake or transport consists of the movement of a substance against a concentration or electrochemical gradient. Often drugs which are similar to a naturally occurring substance are transported by the system intended for that substance (one example is methyldopa which resembles phenylalanine) (86.1).

e) T Some organic anions and cations are secreted in the proximal renal tubule of the kidney by an active carrier mediated mechanism. Many drugs are secreted by systems that secrete naturally occurring substances (86.3).

87 Enzyme inhibition can be a desirable effect or an undesirable side effect of a drug. A knowledge of those agents which may cause enzyme induction or inhibition is definitely desirable.

The following drugs are enzyme inhibitors:
a) phenelzine
b) nitrous oxide
c) isoniazid
d) cinchocaine
e) mercaptopurine

88 A large number of different processes can be responsible for the metabolism of drugs. If you are in any doubt of the completions to this stem read the complete reference section before attempting to answer.

Drugs may be metabolized by:
a) oxidation
b) reduction
c) hydrolysis
d) spontaneous degradation
e) conjugation

References
87.1 Calvery & Williams   p 74–76
87.2 Recent Advances 16   p 19–42
87.3 Goodman & Gilman   p 1148–1149
87.4 Atkinson, Rushman & Lee   p 276

88.1 Calvey & Williams   p 20–24
88.2 Calvey & Williams   p 284–285

87a) T Phenelzine is an inhibitor of monoamine oxidase, the very purpose for which the drug is used therapeutically (87.1).
  b) F Nitrous oxide selectively inhibits vitamin B_{12}. This results in the inhibition of methionine synthetase (87.2).
  c) T Isoniazid inhibits parahydroxylases which normally metabolize anticonvulsants. This effect only reaches significance in so-called slow acetylators (87.3).
  d) T The inhibition of pseudocholinesterase by cinchocaine (often referred to as dibucaine) yields the common index of severity of suxamethonium apnoea. Manufacture of dibucaine has ceased. (87.4).
  e) T Mercaptopurine inhibits phosphoribosylphosphate amidotransferase as quoted in reference (87.1). However, there is a footnote 'enzyme inhibition is dependent on the formation of drug metabolites'. Caution is advocated here. Discretion may be the better part of valour but the recommended response is 'true'.

88a) T Phase 1 reactions include oxidation, often effected by the mixed function oxidase system. A good example here is the conversion of thiopentone to pentobarbitone (88.1).
  b) T Reduction is another phase 1 reaction. An example here is the conversion of chloral hydrate to trichloroethanol (88.1).
  c) T Hydrolysis is the third phase 1 reaction. For example, suxamethonium is hydrolysed to succinate and choline (88.1).
  d) T Atracurium undergoes spontaneous degradation in vivo (the Hoffmann elimination reaction) (88.2). There are not many examples of this process.
  e) T Phase 2 reactions involve the conjugation of other chemical groups with the oxidized, reduced or hydrolysed products of phase 1 reactions (88.1).

89 Halothane is still a mainstay of British anaesthesia despite the widespread fears of possible hepatic damage. Knowledge of this drug must be as extensive as humanly possible. You should be able to quote the physical characteristics of the vapour at will.

Halothane:
a) increases rate of gastric emptying
b) increases cerebral blood flow
c) is metabolized 20%
d) has a MAC of 1.3
e) is excreted renally

90 In any question on neuromuscular blockade first determine the type of blockade being referred to. The terms 'depolarizing', 'non-depolarizing', and 'competitive' may all be used.

Competitive neuromuscular blockade:
a) is antagonized by acidosis
b) is potentiated by hypothermia
c) can be reversed by edrophonium
d) is potentiated by hypocalcaemia
e) occurs after gentamicin administration

References
89.1 Atkinson, Rushman & Lee   p 165–192
89.2 Goodman & Gilman   p 291

90.1 Calvey & Williams   p 281
90.2 Calvey & Williams   p 285–287
90.3 Atkinson, Rushman & Lee   p 282–283

89a) F On the contrary, motility of the gastrointestinal tract is inhibited by halothane (89.1).
   b) T Intracerebral blood flow increases and CSF pressure rises as a direct consequence (89.1). This has led to the cautious use of the agent in the field of neuroanaesthesia although hyperventilation lessens the effect.
   c) T Up to 20% of halothane in body tissue may be degraded but biotransformation is complex. There is both reduction and oxidation depending on circumstances (89.1). It is the reductive pathway of metabolism that is implicated in the vexed area of halothane hepatitis (if such exists).
   d) F The MAC of halothane is 0.75% v/v (89.1).
   e) T There is little renal excretion of halothane. Some 60–80% of absorbed halothane is excreted unchanged in exhaled gas during the first 24 h after administration and smaller amounts will continue to be excreted over the following days or weeks. Of the fraction not exhaled approximately 50% is excreted unchanged via other routes and 50% undergoes biotransformation (89.2).

90a) F The action of the majority of neuromuscular blocking agents is potentiated by acidosis. Gallamine is a notable exception, being antagonized by acidosis. Alcuronium and pancuronium are usually uninfluenced by changes of pH in the physiological range (90.1).
   b) T Hypothermia potentiates competitive neuromuscular blockade (90.1).
   c) T Edrophonium is a short acting anticholinesterase which has gained some popularity in the reversal of competitive neuromuscular blockade (90.2). This has been featured repeatedly in the major UK journals over the last few years.
   d) T Hypocalcaemia and hypermagnesaemia both potentiate competitive neuromuscular blockade (90.3).
   e) T The membrane potential of the end plate is dependent on the presence of calcium and this is reduced by the aminoglycoside antibiotics up to 24 h after administration. This effect is reversed by intravenous calcium but neostigmine is not always efficacious (90.3).

91 Although lithium carbonate is not prescribed by anaesthetists, patients receiving the drug may present for surgery. At first sight of the stem you may feel that you know nothing about lithium but after looking at the completions you may find you know more than you thought.

Lithium carbonate:
a) is used to treat manic depressive psychosis
b) has to be administered by injection
c) has a rapid onset of action
d) has a small therapeutic ratio
e) is actively reabsorbed

92 On reading this stem one would expect to find at least one antimuscarinic drug among the completions and this is so. Some completions here can be deduced from first principles.

The following drugs decrease salivation:
a) orphenadrine
b) promethazine
c) edrophonium
d) dexamphetamine
c) chlorpromazine

References

91.1	Goodman & Gilman	p 418–422
91.2	Vickers, Morgan & Spencer	p 234
92.1	BNF	section 10.2.2
92.2	BNF	section 4.9.2
92.3	BNF	section 3.4.1
92.4	BNF	section 10.2.1
92.5	BNF	section 4.4.2
92.6	BNF	section 4.2.1

91a) T Although it is not a panacea for all forms of cyclothymic illness lithium carbonate is highly effective in the treatment of the manic phase of manic depressive psychosis. Its major effect is that of mood stabilization when used in the long term although it also has a non-specific antidepressant effect (91.1).

b) F Lithium is readily absorbed when given orally. Peak plasma level is usually obtained 2–4 h after ingestion (91.1).

c) F A therapeutic effect is not usually seen until about 3 weeks after continued oral administration (91.3).

d) T The therapeutic ratio of a drug is an index of its effective dose as compared to toxic dose. With respect to lithium a therapeutic effect is seen at plasma concentrations of 0.9–1.4 mmol/l. Plasma levels of 1.5 mmol/l and greater carry no therapeutic benefit and are associated with a greater incidence of unwanted effects, notably fatigue, weakness, slurred speech, ataxia, tremor, nausea, vomiting and diarrhoea, nephrogenic diabetes insipidus, and leucocytosis. In severe toxicity (plasma concentrations greater than 2 mmol/l) muscle rigidity, marked tremor, muscle fasciculations, and epileptic seizures can occur (91.1).

e) T Lithium and sodium are managed by the kidney in a similar fashion. Thus lithium is subject to active reabsorption in the proximal convoluted tubule. 80% of the filtered lithium is reabsorbed (91.1).

92a) T Orphenadrine citrate and hydrochloride belong to the so-called 'centrally acting' group of muscle relaxants. The main uses of the group are in treatment of Parkinson's disease and spasticity. Dry mouth and other antimuscarinic effects are the main side effects (92.1) (92.2).

b) T All the antihistamines, of which promethazine hydrochloride is a classic example, cause antimuscarinic side-effects such as a dry mouth (92.3).

c) F The anticholinesterases, for example neostigmine and edrophonium, increase salivation (92.4). So the reverse is true.

d) T Dexamphetamine is a central nervous system stimulant but does nevertheless cause a dry mouth (92.5).

e) T Antimuscarinic side effects are representative of phenothiazines, chlorpromazine being a typical example of the class (92.6).

93 Antiemetic drugs are encountered frequently in clinical practice. Many questions on this particular class of drugs will relate to their site of action. This is explored in some of the completions below.

Metoclopramide:
a) may cause Parkinsonian symptoms
b) is used to treat duodenal ulcers
c) causes diarrhoea
d) is useful in treating vomiting following radiotherapy
e) is useful in treating motion sickness

94 Clonidine makes frequent and sometimes unwelcome appearances in examinations. The emerging knowledge of presynaptic alpha$_2$ receptors has given the drug an unusually high profile at present, accentuated by knowledge of the adrenergic role in spinal cord transmission.

Clonidine:
a) can cause a dry mouth
b) can cause rebound hypertension on withdrawal
c) is an antagonist at muscarinic receptors
d) can cause drowsiness
e) is used in the treatment of migraine

References

93.1	BNF	section 4.6
93.2	Goodman & Gilman	p 911
93.3	Rang & Dale	p 462–463
93.4	Rang & Dale	p 458
94.1	BNF	section 2.5.2
94.2	Rang & Dale	p 184–185
94.3	Rang & Dale	p 226

93a) T Extrapyramidal effects (Parkinsonian) occur after the administration of metoclopramide especially in children and young adults
given high doses. Procyclidine can be used to abort these Parkinsonian symptoms (93.1). Oculogyric crisis is as painful as it is
distressing to watch.

b) F Metoclopramide increases the rate of gastric emptying which may
possibly be of benefit in gastric ulceration, but its efficacy is poor
in duodenal ulcer patients (93.2).

c) T Diarrhoea is a recognized effect (93.1), probably mediated via a
peripheral action which is, however, not effective in paralytic ileus
(93.3).

d) T Metoclopramide is of value in the treatment of nausea and vomiting associated with uraemia, radiation sickness, anaesthesia, and
gastrointestinal disorders (93.4).

e) F Metoclopramide is ineffective as a treatment for motion sickness
and for vomiting which occurs in labyrinthine disorders (93.4).

94a) T The side effects of clonidine include dry mouth, sedation, depression, fluid retention, bradycardia and Raynaud's phenomenon (94.1).

b) T Sudden withdrawal of clonidine from patients on long-term treatment may cause a hypertensive crisis and this drug must be with-
drawn gradually on a reducing schedule (94.1). In acute use this is
not likely to occur.

c) F Clonidine is an alpha$_2$ selective agonist. It is not firmly established
that its useful effects result from binding to presynaptic alpha$_2$
receptors. There is in fact evidence that its antihypertensive effect
is due to an action on postsynaptic alpha$_2$ receptors in the brain
stem (94.2). This is an evolving issue which is not yet fully
understood.

d) T Side effects of clonidine include dry mouth, sedation, and depression (94.1). For a fuller list see above.

e) T The proven effectiveness of clonidine and propranolol in migraine
is 'hard to explain' (94.3). Say no more.

95 Whilst detailed knowledge of <u>all</u> drugs commonly used in anaesthesia is essential, local anaesthetic agents occur with particular frequency. It is vital to have a thorough understanding of the group and equally important is a knowledge of the toxic doses of each agent with and without added adrenaline.

The following statements are true of lignocaine:
a) it may be given orally to control cardiac arrhythmias
b) it is useful in supraventricular arrhythmias
c) it is an effective local anaesthetic agent if applied to mucous membranes
d) it crosses the blood–brain barrier
e) it is inactivated by plasma cholinesterase

96 Trimetaphan is a drug which may still be used for induced hypotension during anaesthesia although its popularity has declined. A 'bald' stem such as this is not answerable by deduction.

Trimetaphan:
a) is an alpha blocking agent
b) is a ganglion blocking agent
c) reduces cardiac output
d) causes histamine release
e) may be given orally

References	
95.1 BNF	section 2.3
95.2 Rang & Dale	p 755
96.1 Goodman & Gilman	p 793–794
96.2 Goodman & Gilman	p 182–184

95a) F Firstly there is no oral preparation of lignocaine available. Secondly it is essential in acute treatment of arrhythmias that the drug is used intravenously for speed of onset (95.1).

b) F Lignocaine is still used widely for the treatment of ventricular arrhythmias for which it is indicated. It is no help in the treatment of supraventricular arrhythmias (95.1).

c) T Not all local anaesthetic agents will be effective topically on mucous membranes. Lignocaine (along with cocaine) has good tissue penetration and will be effective (95.2). The eutectic mixture of prilocaine and lignocaine (EMLA) is highly effective on mucous membranes.

d) T The basis for the toxicity of local anaesthetic agents is related to their CNS effects and clearly the blood–brain barrier must be permeable to them (95.2).

e) F Lignocaine is an amide linked drug and such drugs are metabolized mainly in the liver. It is ester linked drugs that are inactivated by plasma cholinesterase (95.2). Don't get confused between them.

96a) F Trimetaphan has been used widely to produce hypotension during anaesthesia. It is not an alpha blocking drug but rather belongs to the ganglion blocking group. A particularly useful feature of trimetaphan in hypotensive anaesthesia is its rapid onset and offset when given intravenously. This will obviously give fine control although the profound vasodilatation and hypotension can lead to a troublesome reflex tacyhycardia (96.1).

b) T Trimetaphan is a ganglion blocking agent (96.2). This is the cause of the reduction in arterial pressure.

c) T A fall in cardiac output will occur as a consequence of diminished venous return to the right atrium (preload). This effect is due to the vasodilatation which has been produced by ganglion blockade (96.1).

d) T Trimetaphan is well known to cause histamine release (96.2).

e) F Some ganglion blockers may be given orally but as they are generally quaternary ammonium compounds their absorption from the gastro-intestinal tract is erratic, incomplete, and unpredictable. Additionally, trimetaphan is available in intravenous preparation only—trimetaphan camsylate (96.2).

97 Antibiotics are amongst the more frequently prescribed drugs in the world. They may often be requested by surgeons during induction of anaesthesia. It is recommended that antibiotics are studied in detail, particularly with respect to their specific interactions.

The following drugs are resistant to penicillinase:
a) phenethicillin
b) ampicillin
c) flucloxacillin
d) benzylpenicillin
e) cloxacillin

98 The regulation of blood glucose is normally precisely controlled. There are a number of drugs which interfere with the process which may be a desired or unwanted effect depending on the agent in question.

The following lower blood sugar:
a) adrenaline
b) tolbutamide
c) intravenous alcohol
d) glucagon
e) chlorpropamide

References
97.1 Goodman & Gilman   p 1018–1201
97.2 Goodman & Gilman, 5th edn p 1142
97.3 Goodman & Gilman   p 1076

98.1 Goodman & Gilman   p 196
98.2 Goodman & Gilman   p 1484
98.3 Martindale   p 950
98.4 Goodman & Gilman   p 1488–1489

97a) F Phenethicillin is a cogener of penicillin (the phenoxyethyl analogue of penicillin G). In common with penicillin V it shows exceptional stability in acid media. It is not a member of the penicillinase resistant penicillins (97.2).

b) F Ampicillin is a semisynthetic compound derived from 6-aminopenicillanic acid. It has a wide spectrum of activity but is not resistant to penicillinase (97.3).

c) T Both flucloxacillin and cloxacillin are structurally similar and show marked resistance to cleavage by penicillinase (97.3).

d) F Benzylpenicillin (penicillin G) is susceptible to penicillinase breakdown. It is this feature which led to the search for synthetic derivatives which would be resistant to penicillinase (97.3).

e) T Cloxacillin shows a marked resistance to destruction by penicillinase. This property is logical given the close resemblance of cloxacillin to flucloxacillin which is well known for penicillinase resistance (97.3).

98a) F Adrenaline elevates blood glucose and also reduces the uptake of glucose by peripheral tissues. This is part of the 'fright, flight, and fight' scenario of sympathetic stimulation. Occasionally glycosuria occurs (98.1).

b) T Tolbutamide and chlorpropamide are both sulphonylureas which stimulate islet cells to produce insulin, thereby lowering blood sugar (98.2).

c) T Alcohol has been used as a source of energy in total parenteral nutrition. At higher concentrations the side-effects include: depression of medullary action, lethargy, amnesia, hypothermia, hypoglycaemia (especially in children), stupor, coma, respiratory depression, and cardiovascular collapse (98.3).

d) F Glucagon is a polypeptide hormone produced by the alpha cells of the islets of Langerhans. It increases blood glucose concentration by mobilizing glycogen stored in the liver (98.4).

e) T Chlorpropamide is a common oral hypoglycaemic agent. See b) for detail of its action (98.2).

99 Some completions to this question can be rapidly sourced from your own knowledge while others can be deduced from related facts that you know about the drugs (beware of faulty logic). Some are best considered at length before putting pencil to paper.

The following drugs are active orally:
a) guanethidine
b) pentobarbitone
c) morphine
d) diazepam
e) tubocurarine

100 Heparin is a drug that is used extensively in clinical practice. The action of heparin on the clotting cascade is an interesting topic and a frequent subject of discussion in the examination. Low molecular weight heparins have reached the UK market.

Heparin:
a) activates antithrombin III
b) was the first anticoagulant used clinically
c) is an acidic mucopolysaccharide
d) should not be given intramuscularly
e) has an elimination half life of 1–2 h

References	
99.1 BNF	section 2.5.3
99.2 Calvey & Williams	p 399
99.3 Calvey & Williams	p 314
99.4 Dundee, Clarke & McCaughey	p 188
99.5 Calvey & Williams	p 278
100.1 Rang & Dale	p 387
100.2 Goodman & Gilman	p 1313
100.3 Goodman & Gilman	p 1317
100.4 Rang & Dale	p 386–389

99a) T Guanethidine is an adrenergic neurone blocking drug which is occasionally used for the treatment of moderate to severe hypertension. The recommended starting dose is 10 mg/24 h by mouth (99.1).

b) T Pentobarbitone is the oxygen analogue of thiopentone and is well absorbed orally. It is occasionally used as a premedicant in a dose of 100–200 mg orally 2 h before anaesthesia. Pentobarbitone undergoes extensive distribution and metabolism (99.2).

c) T Morphine is well absorbed from the gastrointestinal tract. It undergoes extensive first pass effects because of its conjugation with glucuronic acid at the 3-hydroxy group. The water soluble complex is excreted in the bile. The subsequent hydrolysis by normal bacterial flora may result in significant entero–hepatic recirculation (99.3).

d) T Diazepam is available in tablet, capsule, and syrup form (99.4). When given orally a maximal effect is seen 60 min after ingestion. There is some evidence to suggest that the oral route is more effective than the intramuscular route (99.4).

e) F The curare drugs were originally used by South American Indians who made crude extracts from plants of the species *Chondodendron*. The extracts were used on blow darts to kill animals for food (99.5). The structure of the non-depolarizing relaxants, all of which are quaternary ammonium compounds, makes them unsuitable for absorption from the intestinal tract.

100a) T Heparan sulphate and heparin are cofactors for antithrombin III. Antithrombin III is an $alpha_2$ globulin which neutralizes thrombin and all the serine proteases in the clotting cascade (X, IX, XI, XII) (100.1).

b) F A phospholipid anticoagulant was first isolated from heart and liver tissue by McLean in 1916. Heparin, named because of its abundance in the liver, was discovered by Howell (1922) in the same laboratory as McLean. The use of heparin in vitro as an anticoagulant 'eventually' led to its use in vivo which was, however, later than the coumarins which predate its clinical use (100.2). The anticoagulant effect in cattle of spoiled sweet clover silage was first described by Schofield in 1924. The causative agent (dicoumarol) was identified in 1939 but the coumarins were thought to be too toxic for human use and were used as rodenticides. In 1951 an army inductee uneventfully survived an attempted suicide using warfarin (100.3).

c) T Heparin is a family of sulphated glycosaminoglycans (mucopolysaccharides) with a range of molecular weights from 4000 to 30 000 Daltons. The molecules are attached to a protein backbone consisting of serine and glycine residues. Heparin is strongly acidic and its anticoagulant activity is related to its electronegative charge (100.4).

d) T Heparin cannot be absorbed from the gastrointestinal tract because of its charge and its large size and is therefore given intravenously or subcutaneously. It is not given intramuscularly because of the possibility of haematoma formation (100.4).

e) F There is immediate onset of action. The half-life of this effect is 40–90 min. Heparin is mainly destroyed by hepatic heparinase although platelet factor IV also has the capacity to neutralize it (100.4).

101 Clarify in your mind the differences between spontaneous muscle movements and epileptiform activity on the EEG. This is relevant with regard to etomidate and methohexitone, for example.

The following drugs are contraindicated in patients receiving anticonvulsant therapy:
a) suxamethonium
b) thiopentone
c) halothane
d) methohexitone
e) ketamine

102 The kinins are an elusive family which may become lost in a busy schedule of revision. Unless your knowledge of bradykinin is extensive this question will prove to be impossible to answer without risk. The final completion is unwelcome as it poses three separate questions in one.

Bradykinin:
a) causes contraction of the uterus
b) may be injected into the cerebral ventricles without effect
c) causes bronchoconstriction in asthmatics
d) is metabolized in the lung
e) stimulates nerve endings to cause pain, which is blocked by aspirin through a peripheral action

References

101.1 Vickers, Morgan & Spencer	p 112
101.2 Vickers, Morgan & Spencer	p 135
101.3 Vickers, Morgan & Spencer	p 142–144
101.4 Atkinson, Rushman & Lee	p 237
101.5 Dundee & Wyant	p 155
101.6 Dundee & Wyant	p 240
102.1 Rang & Dale	p 274
102.2 Wall & Melzack	p 190–198
102.3 Nunn	p 290
102.4 Rang & Dale	p 710

101a) F Suxamethonium is the relaxant of choice in preventing the peripheral motor manifestations of the induced nervous discharge in electroconvulsive treatment. There is no direct effect on either convulsant activity or anticonvulsant drugs (101.1).

b) F Thiopentone and diazepam are recommended for use in the treatment of convulsions. However, these drugs do cause brain stem depression which may be cumulative with any other anticonvulsants that are being concomitantly administered (101.1).

c) F Halothane produces marked central nervous system depression (101.2). It is enflurane that produces central stimulant actions in which it differs from other inhalational agents. Seizures have been reported up to 1 week after enflurane anaesthesia, but under conditions of normocapnia enflurane does not exacerbate pre-existing epileptic activity (101.3).

d) F Answer this at your peril! Methohexitone has been found to cause abnormal spike discharges in epileptic subjects. It does not suppress epileptic manifestations and may be implicated in the aetiology of fits (101.4). Because of the risk of extravascular injection of thiopentone, methohexitone has been recommended for use as an anticonvulsant! (101.5). It has been suggested that of the four isomers of methohexitone, two have depressant CNS effects while two are excitatory.

e) F Anticonvulsant drugs are not a contraindication to ketamine. It would not be the most suitable drug to use under most circumstances (101.6).

102a) T Bradykinin is spasmogenic for several types of smooth muscle including that of the intestine, uterus, and bronchial system. The contraction is slow and sustained. It is also a very potent vasodilator (102.1).

b) F Receptors within cerebral ventricles respond markedly to bradykinin. Their function as nocioceptors is uncertain (102.2).

c) T Spasm of the bronchial smooth muscle results in bronchoconstriction (102.1) which may be severe.

d) T Bradykinin is very effectively removed during passage through the lung and other vascular beds. The half life varies between 4 and 17 s. ACE (angiotensin converting enzyme) appears to be the enzyme responsible (102.3).

e) T The pain caused by kinins is relieved by aspirin and other members of the NSAIDs. Bradykinin activates the prostaglandin system and it is this which results in pain. Aspirin inhibits prostaglandin synthesis peripherally (102.4).

103 It might be assumed when reading both these stems concerning drugs that are used every day that it will be possible to answer all the completions. Be cautious. This may not be so despite their familiarity. Anaesthetic gases and vapours have a very high examination profile.

Nitrous oxide:
a) increases cardiac output
b) decreases peripheral resistance
c) causes no significant change in arterial blood pressure
d) has a blood gas partition coefficient less than 0.5
e) sensitizes the heart to exogenous catecholamines

104 Not a day goes by in any operating theatre in the land without a bottle of halothane being opened. Are you confident that you know the drug you are using every day? Try this.

Halothane:
a) has a greater respiratory depressant effect than isoflurane
b) is an halogenated ether
c) raises intracranial pressure
d) increases cerebral metabolism
e) causes cerebral vasoconstriction in the presence of hyperventilation

References
103.1 Dundee, Clarke & McCaughey   p 127–131
103.2 Goodman & Gilman   p 298–300
103.3 Recent Advances 16   p 23

104.1 Goodman & Gilman   p 295
104.2 Calvey & Williams   p 210
104.3 Vicker, Morgan & Spencer   p 135–141
104.4 Current Anaesthesia and Critical
          Care (1990) 1.2   p 79
104.5 Nunn   p 463

103a) F Although various sources differ on the degree, the consensus view states that nitrous oxide causes a fall in cardiac output (103.1) due to a direct myocardial depressant action. A sympathomimetic action mediated centrally may ameliorate this effect. Myocardial contractility is depressed in vivo (103.2).

b) F In addition to sensitizing vascular smooth muscle to circulating noradrenaline, levels of circulating noradrenaline are increased. Nitrous oxide increases peripheral resistance and raises mean arterial pressure when used with halothane in vivo. This is despite the cardiac output effect described above (103.2).

contrary?

c) F There is a rise in blood pressure as described above (103.2).

d) T The blood gas partition coefficient of nitrous oxide is 0.47 at 37°C (103.2).

e) F The authors can only quote from a recent review of nitrous oxide: 'The possibility that nitrous oxide may increase the sensitivity of the heart to exogenous catecholamines does not appear to have been investigated' (103.3).

104a) F MAC for MAC, which is the only logical way of comparing volatile agents, isoflurane has a more profound depressant effect on respiration than halothane. Pa_{CO_2} rises to about the same level but the ventilatory response is depressed more with isoflurane (104.1).

b) F Halothane is an halogenated hydrocarbon. It is not an ether because it has no etheric bond (104.2).

c) T Halothane is well known to increase both cerebral blood flow and intracranial pressure, an effect which it shares with the other commonly used volatile agents (104.3).

d) F Halothane in the order of 1 MAC or so will cause a decrease in CMR_{O_2} of 26% (104.4).

e) F This completion deliberately sets out to mislead. Although halothane may not show its cerebral vasodilating effects under hyperventilation, nevertheless the characteristic feature of the agent is not vasoconstriction but vasodilatation. Be on your guard! (104.5).

105 Muscle relaxants of all categories are commonplace in practice. The more recently introduced agents such as atracurium and vecuronium are becoming evergreen topics. It is probable that it will not be long before they are joined by mivacurium and doxacurium.

Atracurium
a) is metabolized by Hoffmann degradation and alkaline ester hydrolysis
b) is metabolized more rapidly if temperature is increased
c) is metabolized more rapidly in acidosis
d) contains benzenesulfonic acid
e) causes systemic histamine release

106 Vecuronium, an even more recent addition to the anaesthetist's armamentarium than atracurium, provides a topical subject particularly in pharmacology vivas. Be prepared to be questioned on the comparative merits of the non-depolarizing agents with respect to their pharmacological properties. It is interesting to note that vecuronium and atracurium are the two most popular drugs in this group in the UK according to SOAP (Survey of Anaesthetic Practice).

Vecuronium:
a) is a monoquaternary compound
b) has a shorter duration than pancuronium
c) is stable in water
d) is mainly excreted in bile
e) crosses the placenta

References

105.1 Miller	p 402–403
105.2 Data Sheet Compendium	p 1739
105.3 Trissel	p 76
105.4 Miller	p 408
106.1 Dundee, Clarke & McCaughey	p 306–307
106.2 Atkinson, Rushman & Lee	p 267
106.3 Atkinson, Rushman & Lee	p 270
106.4 Concise Oxford English Dictionary	p 1115
106.5 Data Sheet Compendium	p 1064

105a) T The metabolism of atracurium occurs by Hoffmann degradation and alkaline ester hydrolysis both in the plasma and elsewhere in the body. The Hoffmann elimination pathway is characterized by the spontaneous breakdown of atracurium under physiological conditions to yield mainly inactive fragments (laudanosine and pentamethylene-1,5-diacrylate). The degree of neuromuscular blockade produced by laudanosine is the subject of much debate. It is probably of little significance clinically. In summary the metabolism of atracurium is complicated and not yet completely resolved (105.1).

b) F Variations in body temperature and pH of the patient within the physiological range will not significantly alter the duration of action of atracurium (105.2). In deliberate hypothermia the duration of action is markedly prolonged (105.1).

c) F Changes within physiological pH range do not change metabolic rate (105.1).

d) T Atracurium is supplied as the besylate salt in vials with benzene-sulfonic acid as a pH adjuster to keep the pH between 3.25 and 3.65 (105.3).

e) T Although this effect is mild, both atracurium and vecuronium cause some systemic histamine release. Atracurium may also cause local histamine release at the site of injection (105.4). This can occasionally be alarmingly obvious from the weals which appear on the patient's arm.

106a) T Vecuronium is the monoquaternary homologue of pancuronium and the two have very much in common (106.1). One of the quaternary nitrogen groups was deliberately removed from the pancuronium molecule in an attempt to prevent cardiac effects, since this was thought to be the group responsible. The other quaternary nitrogen group is responsible for the blocking property of the molecule.

b) T When considering two relaxants the comparison must be made between comparable doses, e.g. ED95. With respect to the two drugs here vecuronium has a shorter duration than pancuronium on that basis. The duration of vecuronium is 10–20 min (106.2) and of pancuronium 20–30 min (106.3).

c) F Vecuronium is stable in water to the degree that a solution once made up will remain active for 24 h at room temperature (106.2). Deacetylation of the molecule at position three of the steroid nucleus starts after reconstitution. Normally to aid shelf life a buffered lyophilized cake is supplied. The definition of stable is 'not easily changed or destroyed or altered in value' (106.4).

d) T Biliary excretion is the major route of excretion (106.5) for vecuronium.

e) F There is no transfer of vecuronium across the placenta (106.2).

107 Edrophonium has recently come under the spotlight within the specialty. The reason for this will be apparent in the discussion section following this question.

The following statements are true of edrophonium:
a) dilates the pupil
b) has a long duration of action
c) may be used to reverse competitive neuromuscular block
d) causes muscle weakness
e) crosses the blood–brain barrier

108 There is little defence against such a wide ranging question on infrequent side effects of a variety of drugs. Do not attempt to answer those items of which you are uncertain. It is unlikely that you will be able to say for sure that any one of these does <u>not</u> cause agranulocytosis. A safer approach may therefore be to pick the ones which do and then leave it at that.

The following cause agranulocytosis:
a) nitrous oxide
b) aspirin
c) carbimazole
d) chlorpropamide
e) chloramphenicol

References	
107.1 Rang & Dale	p 177
107.2 Rang & Dale	p 173–174
107.3 Miller	p 419
107.4 Goodman & Gilman	p 140
107.5 Goodman & Gilman	p 137
108.1 Recent Advances 16	p 32
108.2 Goodman & Gilman	p 648
108.3 Data Sheet Compendium	p 1005
108.4 Data Sheet Compendium	p 1133
108.5 Data Sheet Compendium	p 1104

107a) T Edrophonium is an anticholinesterase. The principal use of these drugs in glaucoma is that of pupillary constriction which aids aqueous drainage (107.1).

b) F Edrophonium belongs to the short acting class of anticolinesterases. Binding occurs only to the anionic site of cholinesterase and the ionic bond formed is weak and readily reversible. This is responsible for its evanescent action (in the order of minutes) (107.2).

c) T Edrophonium, along with neostigmine and pyridostigmine, has been used extensively in reversing competitive neuromuscular block. There is a more rapid onset of action and reduced atropine requirements compared with neostigmine (107.3). It is this role of edrophonium which has received such a wealth of attention recently.

d) T As a consequence of the nicotinic action of edrophonium at the neuromuscular junction of skeletal muscle, generalized muscle weakness occurs (107.4).

e) F In common with the other anticholinesterases edrophonium is a quaternary ammonium compound which does not readily cross the blood–brain barrier (107.5).

108a) T Administration of nitrous oxide, even at low concentrations, will cause leucopenia within 3 days and agranulocytosis in 5–7 days. Recovery of bone marrow occurs within 4 days of withdrawal. Vitamin B_{12} treatment has no effect (108.1).

b) F Salicylates do not ordinarily alter the white cell count except for a therapeutic reduction in acute rheumatic fever (108.2).

c) T Bone marrow depression is a recognized effect of carbimazole and may lead on to agranulocytosis (108.3). Regular white cell counts are recommended for patients receiving the drug long term.

d) T Although relatively uncommon, leucopenia and agranulocytosis are well documented side-effects (108.4) after treatment with chlorpropamide.

e) T Chloramphenicol is well known to cause agranulocytosis and in addition aplastic anaemia has been reported (108.5). This unfortunate sequel may occur after relatively trivial exposure to the drug.

109 The various physical properties of the common anaesthetic vapours are fair game in a pharmacology examination. Guessing in this type of question is particularly suicidal. Only answer the completions that you know and be very wary of the range of figures which may occur in different sources for values of partition coefficients, MAC, boiling points, and the like. Blood gas partition coefficients are usually measured and quoted at body temperature. Such a fact has, unfortunately, to be assumed in this question.

The following agents have blood gas partition coefficients less than 2:
a) halothane
b) enflurane
c) methoxyflurane
d) diethyl ether
e) isoflurane

110 Comparative questions on vapours appear with some regularity. It can be quite difficult to obtain factual information on the relative effects of the common vapours and readers are invited to study the references for detail.

Enflurane:
a) is more potent than halothane
b) depresses cardiac output more than halothane
c) is metabolized to fluoride ions
d) is an halogenated hydrocarbon
e) is flammable in oxygen

References

109.1 Dundee, Clarke & McCaughey   p 99
109.2 Vickers, Morgan & Spencer   p 124

110.1 Dundee, Clarke & McCaughey   p 105–106
110.2 Nimmo & Smith   p 44–45
110.3 Vickers, Morgan & Spencer   p 142–144
110.4 Vickers, Morgan & Spencer   p 157–159
110.5 Atkinson, Rushman & Lee   p 192

109 For purely factual recall exercises like this it is useful to have your own revision table for the physical properties of the common anaesthetic gases and vapours. An amalgamation of those in references (109.1) and (109.2) would be ideal.

a) F The blood gas coefficient of an anaesthetic vapour gives an idea of its speed of onset and also speed of offset (or recovery). In general, agents with lower blood gas solubilities are faster acting and have shorter recovery times. This applies usefully to halothane when compared to isoflurane. The figure for halothane is 2.3 and that for isoflurane 1.4 (109.1).

b) T Although the oft-quoted figure for enflurane of 1.8 is a bit too close for comfort (109.2).

c) F The blood gas coefficient for methoxyflurane is 12. Although no longer in clinical use methoxyflurane still makes regular guest appearances (109.2).

d) F The figure for diethyl ether is 12 (109.1).

e) T Isoflurane has a blood gas coefficient of 1.4 (109.1).

110a) F MAC is a good indicator of relative potency for the inhalational agents. The lower the MAC value the more potent is the agent. The relative values are 0.75% v/v for halothane and 1.68% v/v for enflurane. Thus enflurane has approximately half the potency of halothane (110.1). Volumetric percentage is a useful measure of vapour concentration as it enables comparisons to be made between gases and true vapours.

b) F Initial work suggested that enflurane was a much more profound negative inotrope than either halothane or isoflurane. Experimentally it had been difficult to administer more than 2 MAC enflurane due to its effects on cardiac output. Now it is generally accepted that enflurane has less negative inotropic effect than halothane but more than isoflurane (110.2).

c) T The most important product of enflurane metabolism is fluoride. Although absolute levels depend on MAC-hour dose levels, generally serum fluoride levels reach a maximum of 25 μmol/l (110.3).

d) F Enflurane is an halogenated ethyl–methylether and also an isomer of isoflurane (110.4).

e) T Concentrations of enflurane greater than 4.25% are flammable in 20% oxygen in nitrous oxide (110.5). Clinically such concentrations are not frequently used.

111 Chlorpromazine, infrequently encountered in mainstream anaesthesia, exhibits a wide spectrum of different pharmacological actions. Some of these effects are examined below.

Side effects of chlorpromazine include:
a) hypothermia
b) photosensitivity
c) hiccoughs
d) sedation
e) jaundice

112 An extension of the previous question. Haloperidol is an agent which is frequently compared with chlorpromazine. Although both agents have similar actions the respective emphasis of these is different.

In comparison with chlorpromazine, haloperidol has:
a) less sedative effect
b) more anticholinergic effect
c) less extrapyramidal effect
d) longer duration of action
e) lower risk of oculogyric crisis

References
111.1 Dundee, Clarke & McCaughey   p 195–196
111.2 BNF   section 4.2.1

112.1 Goodman & Gilman   p 386–401
112.2 Goodman & Gilman   p 1669
112.3 Goodman & Gilman   p 1683

111a) T One of the commonest effects of chlorpromazine is alpha receptor blockade. This inevitably leads to vasodilatation and accompanying heat loss. An effect on temperature regulation by the depression of the temperature regulating centre and reduction of shivering exacerbate this (111.1). The reduction in muscle tone will contribute to this effect.

b) T Photosensitivity is but one of a whole host of unwanted effects varying from the trivial, such as nasal congestion, to lethal agranulocytosis. A full list may be found in BNF (111.2).

c) F Far from being an unwanted effect this is an indication for treatment with chlorpromazine although reports of its effectiveness vary (111.2).

d) T Chlorpromazine is a powerful sedative and finds extensive use in violent psychotic patients (111.1).

e) T Jaundice is a potentially serious side effect. It is reported to occur in 0.5% of treated patients. The picture is that of cholestatic jaundice often accompanied by eosinophilia and fever (111.1).

112a) T Haloperidol is not noted for profound sedation whereas chlorpromazine certainly is (111.2). That is one of the most marked differences between the two agents.

b) F Haloperidol has very little anticholinergic effect (112.1).

c) F There is a high incidence of extrapyramidal side effects with haloperidol especially in younger patients (112.1). These manifestations are usually either oculogyric crisis or full opisthotonus, both of which are painful and alarming.

d) F Although onset times are similar the half life of chlorpromazine is longer. The values for each are chlorpromazine 30 h (112.2) and haloperidol 18 h (112.3).

e) F Oculogyric crises are more frequent with haloperidol as are other abnormalities of motor activity (112.1).

Haloperidol: extrapyramidal more S/E
shorter duration
less sedation
less anticholinergic effects

113 Phenytoin is not only a drug that is frequently encountered as inter-current medication in patients presenting for surgery but also one that serves to illustrate important pharmacokinetic principles. It is doubtless these that lead to its regular inclusion in the MCQ paper.

Phenytoin:
a) has a high therapeutic ratio
b) can induce microsomal enzymes
c) can exhibit first order elimination kinetics
d) can exhibit zero order elimination kinetics
e) exhibits a constant half life over its whole therapeutic dose range

114 Bromocriptine is useful in the treatment of acromegaly and the suppression of lactation. The drug has a use in Parkinson's disease in patients who are intolerant of levodopa. Unfortunately it has several unwanted effects.

Bromocriptine:
a) is a dopamine receptor agonist
b) can cause infertility
c) can be reversed by chlorpromazine
d) has useful antiemetic properties
e) can cause pleural effusions

References

113.1 BNF	section 4.8.1
113.2 Vickers, Morgan & Spencer	p 113–115
113.3 Goodman & Gilman	p 1700
114.1 Rang & Dale	p 581–583
114.2 BNF	section 6.7.1

113a) F Phenytoin has a narrow therapeutic index and the relationship between dose and plasma concentration is non-linear so that monitoring of plasma levels greatly assists dosage adjustment (113.1).

b) T Metabolism is influenced by hepatic microsomal enzyme induction and phenytoin itself causes this effect (113.2).

c) T In the initial stages of phenytoin treatment when plasma levels are below 10 µg/ml, first order kinetics apply. That is to say, the excretion of the drug varies exponentially with its plasma level. At higher concentrations, even in the presence of enzyme induction, which has a finite value, the excretion kinetics change to zero order because the excretion pathway becomes saturated. Zero order kinetics are typical of drugs like alcohol and the rate of excretion in this instance is fixed and does not vary with plasma concentrations (113.2). It is this pattern of excretion kinetics that causes this drug to appear so frequently in the examination. Watch out for this in the vivas. Be prepared.

d) T Zero order kinetics only apply to phenytoin after saturation. This completion is nonetheless true because the drug <u>can</u> exhibit zero order kinetics on occasion (113.2). Saturation kinetics is a concept which is often asked in the examination and phenytoin is a useful example to quote.

e) F The half life will not be constant if more than one order of kinetics applies over the therapeutic dose range (113.2). The half life is between 6 and 24 h (113.3).

114a) T Bromocriptine is a partial agonist at D_1 receptors and an agonist at D_2 receptors. For futher information the reader is referred to Rang & Dale (114.1).

b) F Bromocriptine is a recognized treatment for infertility (114.2).

c) T Phenothiazines are antagonists at D_1 and D_2 receptors and will reverse the dopaminergic actions of bromocriptine (114.1). This effect may have clinical importance if phenothiazines are administered to patients receiving treatment with bromocriptine.

d) F Like apomorphine, bromocriptine is an agonist at dopaminergic receptors and is liable as a consequence to have emetic properties rather than the reverse (114.1).

e) T In high doses pleural effusions occur and these may be so severe as to necessitate the withdrawal of treatment (114.2).

115 No revision book for this examination is complete without a stock of material that relates to the tricyclic antidepressants. This question is more clinically based than some that may be encountered. It is typical of the genre.

In poisoning with tricyclic antidepressants:
a) skin blisters occur in the unconscious patient
b) little benefit is to be gained by gastric lavage more than 12 h after ingestion
c) charcoal haemoperfusion is the treatment of choice
d) acute liver necrosis follows rapidly
e) cardiac dysrhythmias are a serious problem

116 Do not risk any guesses here because the answers may be surprising. Currently vancomycin is the drug of choice for treating antibiotic-associated pseudomembranous colitis (116.1).

Antibiotics shown to precipitate pseudomembranous colitis in humans include:
a) clindamycin
b) cephalothin
c) metronidazole
d) ampicillin
e) gentamicin

References		
115.1 Goodman & Gilman	p 413	
115.2 Dunnill & Colvin	p 227	
116.1 BNF	section 5.1.7	
116.2 BNF	section 5.1.6	
116.3 BNF	section 5.1.2	
116.4 BNF	section 5.1.11	
116.5 BNF	section 5.1.1.3	
116.6 BNF	section 5.1.4	

115a) F Although skin rashes and photosensitization do occur, skin blisters are not a reported occurrence in acute poisoning (115.1).

b) T The absorption of tricyclic antidepressants is rapid and complete from the gastrointestinal tract. Gastric lavage is considered useful in antidepressant poisoning if the overdose was taken within 8–10 h of reaching medical attention (115.2).

c) F Haemoperfusion is not effective and is not recommended. Diuresis is equally useless (115.1).

d) F Although liver damage may occur as a late result, it is not seen in early cases (115.1).

e) T The tricyclics are well known for their propensity to cause cardiac arrhythmias, and monitoring of the ECG is most highly recommended (115.1).

116a) T Clindamycin is a classic example of an antibiotic which will cause pseudomembranous colitis as did its predecessor lincomycin (116.2).

b) T Although a rare event after treatment with cephalothin, nonetheless pseudomembranous colitis has been reported (116.3).

c) F Metronidazole has not been reported to precipitate this effect in humans. Note that metronidazole itself is effective in the treatment of pseudomembranous colitis! (116.4).

d) T This is not a common association but it has been reported (116.5).

e) T A reported association exists between gentamicin therapy and pseudomembranous colitis (116.6).

117 The anticoagulants illustrate a great deal of pharmacology and physiology. They rightly deserve to appear again in this volume. Coumarins, heparin, or ancrod may be subjects in MCQ or viva format. Remember that the physiology of clotting is liable to be examined as well.

Warfarin:
a) has no clinical effect for 36 h after a single dose
b) may be reversed by protamine
c) is highly protein bound
d) is effective in vitro
e) interferes with the action of vitamin K

118 It is remarkably easy to confuse the two main classes of anticoagulants. These two questions have been deliberately juxtaposed to aid clarity of thought.

Heparin:
a) is a mucopolysaccharide
b) carries a strongly negative ionic charge
c) may be given by a variety of routes
d) affects antithrombin III
e) has a long half life

References	
117.1 BNF	section 2.8.2
117.2 Goodman & Gilman	p 1317–1319
118.1 Dundee, Clarke & McCaughey	p 441–442
118.2 Vickers, Morgan & Spencer	p 452–455
118.3 BNF	section 2.8.1
118.4 Goodman & Gilman	p 1317–1319
118.5 Goodman & Gilman	p 1683

117a) T Because it acts on vitamin K, no effect will be seen after a first dose of warfarin for 36–48 h. Clinically this is the 'loading' dose. Subsequent regular dosage must be controlled by clotting tests, e.g. International Normalized Ratio (INR). For an immediate effect heparin is the only choice (117.1).

b) F Protamine sulphate is the reversal agent for heparin. Warfarin acts by interfering with the synthesis of the vitamin K-dependent clotting factors. The hepatic manufacture of factors II, VII, IX, and X is reduced by a competitive inhibition of vitamin K. Thus the only logical reversal of coumarins is vitamin K itself (117.2).

c) T Warfarin is almost completely protein bound to albumin although this binding is weak (117.2).

d) F Unlike heparin the coumarins are not active in vitro (117.2).

e) T Warfarin is a vitamin K antagonist (117.2). That is the basis of its anticoagulant effect.

118a) T Heparin is not a single substance. It is a mixture of mucopolysaccharides obtained from porcine intestinal mucosa or beef lung. The commercial preparation is a mixture with molecular weights between 5000 and 35 000 Daltons. Purer low molecular weight heparins are currently appearing on the market for the first time (118.1).

b) T It is thought that the basis of action of heparin is partly related to its strong electronegative charge (118.2).

c) T Heparin is mostly used by bolus or intravenous infusion but has a clinical use by subcutaneous injection for the prophylaxis of deep venous thrombosis after surgery (118.3). Heparin can be given intramuscularly but larger doses are required, the response is slower, the injections are painful and there is a tendency to haematomas at the site of injection (118.2). This is not a recommended route.

d) T Heparin inhibits factors involved in the conversion of prothrombin to thrombin. This is accomplished by the facilitation of the formation of antithrombin III with each of the four activated proteases of the clotting cascade, activated factors IX, X, XI, and XII (118.4).

e) F The half life is quoted as $26 + (0.323 \times \text{dose}) \pm 12$ min! The dose is measured in IU/kg. Translated—the half life of heparin is dose dependent (possibly due to saturation kinetics with end product inhibition). In essence the half life is based on 26 min with a dose-dependent addition. This does not constitute a long half life (118.5).

119 Malignant hyperpyrexia is not seen commonly in anaesthetic practice. Despite this, both the condition and its treatment have a high profile in all the anaesthetic examinations. Dantrolene is essential subject matter for any anaesthetic revision text (see Question 12).

Dantrolene sodium:
a) is a skeletal muscle relaxant
b) is coloured orange
c) is supplied mixed with mannitol
d) has vasodilating effects
e) is a calcium antagonist

120 Naloxone is an agent with the most intriguing range of effects outside its famous role as a reversal agent for opioid overdose (122.1).

Naloxone will reverse the respiratory depression of the following:
a) methadone
b) halothane
c) dihydrocodeine
d) midazolam
e) meptazinol

References

119.1 Data Sheet Compendium		p 1018
119.2 Vickers, Morgan & Spencer		p 265
119.3 Miller		p 949
120.1 BJA (1985) 57		p 547–550
120.2 Goodman & Gilman		p 514–517
120.3 BNF		section 15.1.7
120.4 Goodman & Gilman		p 514

119a) T Dantrolene is the recommended treatment for malignant hyperpyrexia. It has other clinical indications, for example in spastic conditions for the relief of muscle spasm. This is due to a skeletal muscle relaxant effect. Dantrolene produces a dissociation of excitation–contraction coupling by an effect on calcium release within the sarcoplasmic reticulum (119.1). The site of this action is thought to be on the transverse tubular sarcoplasmic reticulum coupling.

b) T In intravenous form, dantrolene is supplied as a powder for reconstitution which is orange (119.2).

c) T Dantrolene itself has a low water solubility (but high lipid solubility) and is supplied as a lyophilized sodium salt together with mannitol in the same vial (119.2).

d) F Although some experimental evidence has pointed to an association between cardiovascular collapse and therapeutic doses of dantrolene, the relevance of this to man has not been established (119.1).

e) F This phrase is generally taken to refer to calcium channel blocking agents. The calcium antagonists act primarily on surface membranes of cardiac or smooth muscle, whereas the efficacy of dantrolene is related to calcium release from the sarcoplasmic reticulum (119.3).

120a) T Methadone is a partial agonist at opioid receptors. Its major use is in treatment of opioid dependence. Naloxone will reverse the respiratory depression of any opioid agonist or partial agonist if given in sufficient doses (120.2).

b) F Naloxone will not reverse the respiratory depressant effects of non-opioid agents (120.3). For interest, in the cat, the respiratory depression caused by halothane has been reversed by naloxone when perfused into the fourth ventricle.

c) T Dihydrocodeine is an opioid and is thus reversible by naloxone (120.2).

d) F Benzodiazepines have their own specific antidote. This is the benzodiazepine receptor antagonist flumazenil (120.3).

e) T This is true but it must be stated that as meptazinol does not behave entirely in a similar manner to other opioids the reversal may not be complete (120.4). At the time of writing there is some residual uncertainty as to the exact site of action of meptazinol.

121 There are several pulmonary reflexes of varying importance. One that crops up more than most is the Hering–Breuer reflex, especially with regard to its relevance to human physiology. There has been recent controversy over this issue and readers are referred to BJA (121.1).

The Hering–Breuer reflex:
a) is not seen in man
b) may help to inflate the neonatal lung
c) is mediated via the vagus
d) is a primitive reflex
e) consists of a sudden inspiratory gasp

122 Hypoxia has a vasoconstricting effect on the pulmonary circulation which is the opposite effect to that on the systemic vasculature. Hypoxic pulmonary vasoconstriction is an important means of diverting flow from regions of low oxygen tension. Learn the agents which abolish the reflex response.

Hypoxic pulmonary vasoconstriction:
a) occurs in response to lowered Pa_{O_2}
b) is mediated via the vagus
c) is more marked in respiratory acidosis
d) is a cause of true shunt
e) is abolished by inhalational agents

References
121.1 BJA (1991) 66	p 627–628
121.2 Nunn	p 92–93
122.1 Nunn	p 127–128
122.2 West	p 54–55
122.3 Nunn	p 376

121a) T Many students have been assured of the validity of the Hering–Breuer reflex in man. This is the misplaced extrapolation of animal work to the human. The reflex is very weak in man, if not absent. The correct response is therefore controversial. Hering and Breuer were two different men (121.2).

b) F This refers to the neonatal 'gasp reflex'. Although it has not been established whether the 'gasp reflex' of the newborn infant is analogous to Head's paradoxical reflex, it is <u>not</u> the Hering–Breuer reflex (122.1).

c) T Afferents from all pulmonary receptors are conducted via the vagus. Some may be additionally carried in the sympathetic chain (121.2).

d) T This reflex occurs in animals and neonates. It is classified as a primitive reflex which may once have had some advantage teleologically speaking (121.2).

e) F The Hering–Breuer reflex consists of inhibition of inspiration in response to a sustained inflation of the lung. In contrast, a sudden inspiratory gasp is Head's paradoxical reflex (121.2).

122a) T Pulmonary vasoconstriction is mediated primarily by the alveolar Po_2 but also by the pulmonary arterial Po_2 (122.1).

b) F Some pulmonary vasoconstriction may result from hypoxic stimulation of the peripheral chemoreceptors by way of sympathetic efferent pathways but this is less important than the local effect, which can also operate in the isolated lung (122.1).

c) T Hypercapnia has a slight pressor effect and reinforces hypoxic vasoconstriction probably by causing acidosis (122.1).

d) F Shunt refers to blood which enters the arterial system without going through ventilated areas of the lung (122.2). Hypoxic pulmonary vasoconstriction will reduce the amount of blood taking such a course and so will reduce shunt (122.1) (122.3).

e) T Inhalational agents depress hypoxic pulmonary vasoconstriction *if* an allowance is made for changes in cardiac output. However, intravenous induction agents have no effect (122.3). In general it is fair to say that the effects of inhalational agents are subject to some controversy.

123 Although a neglected area of study the skin has several different physiological roles. It is wise to include lesser topics in revision if scheduling allows.

The functions of the skin include:
a) thermoregulation
b) nociception
c) phagocytosis
d) sodium excretion
e) melanin production

124 Blood transfusion is not without problems. There are data sheets for blood products which provide a great deal of useful revision material. Usually these will be available in the haematology department of every hospital.

The transfusion of stored blood:
a) may cause leucocytosis
b) may cause rigors
c) may result in pyrexia
d) may reduce 2,3-DPG
e) may cause hypokalaemia

References

123.1 Guyton   p 805
123.2 Ganong   p 107
123.3 Guyton   p 368
123.4 Guyton   p 800–801
123.5 Guyton   p 851

124.1 Nimmo & Smith   p 388–392
124.2 Nunn   p 266–267
124.3 Atkinson, Rushman & Lee   p 821–824

123a) T There is both a local element and a hypothalamic element to the thermoregulation mediated via the skin. This occurs by alterations in the state of vasodilatation and vasoconstriction (123.1).

b) T Some authorities draw a distinction between pain receptors and nociceptors. Nevertheless nociceptors are naked nerve endings within the skin which respond to noxious stimuli (123.2).

c) T Although the skin usually provides an impenetrable barrier, in the presence of active infection macrophages divide and phagocytose foreign particles (123.3).

d) T Sweat contains between 5 mmol/l and 60 mmol/l of sodium (123.4). Sweating is a method of sodium excretion but it is obligatory.

e) T Melanin is produced by melanocytes between the dermis and epidermis (123.5).

124a) T Contamination of stored blood with infective agents can occur although it is fortunately rare. Both contamination and a mild ABO type incompatibility reaction will lead to a raised white cell count (124.1).

b) T This is not a very common occurrence. The incidence of rigors is around 1% of transfusions (124.1).

c) T As described above, both infective agents and incompatibility reactions may contribute to a pyrexial response (124.1).

d) T 2,3-DPG is 2,3-diphosphoglycerate. The level of 2,3-DPG falls with time of storage. In ACD (acid–citrate–dextrose) preserved blood 2,3-DPG levels fall to zero. CPD (citrate–phosphate–dextrose) preserved blood on the other hand reduces the rate of 2,3-DPG depletion. Transfusion of blood with low levels of 2,3-DPG reduces, by a diluent effect, total red cell 2,3-DPG. This contributes to a left shift of the oxygen dissociation curve (124.2).

e) F The potassium level approaches 30 mmol/l in stored blood toward the end of the shelf life. Potassium intoxication can result during or shortly after blood transfusion especially in the presence of metabolic acidosis. Hyperkalaemia is usually transient as potassium will re-enter the cells (124.3).

125 Clinically based questions can prove difficult to answer especially if there is an element of opinion involved. The question below concerns a straightforward clinical situation and should present little problem.

A pregnant woman of blood group A Pos. can safely be given 500 ml of:
a) group A neg. whole blood
b) blood containing dextrose
c) blood with no effective white cells
d) blood containing 14 mmol/l potassium
e) blood which has been stored at −4°C for some weeks

126 Acid-base balance is often a topic in the viva situation. It will pay to make sure that the various terms involved are fully understood. The ITU ward round provides a good opportunity to examine the topic with a mentor.

The standard bicarbonate:
a) is raised in metabolic alkalosis
b) is raised in respiratory acidosis
c) indicates the respiratory component of acid base
d) is the base excess at $P\text{co}_2$ 5.3 kPa
e) is the same as standard base excess

References
125.1 Atkinson, Rushman & Lee   p 819
125.2 Scurr, Feldman & Soni   p 466–472
125.3 Nimmo & Smith   p 381

126.1 Davenport   p 116–122

125a) T The essence of this question is centred on Rhesus (Rh) grouping and its importance in women and those who may require further transfusion. Pregnancy is not an important factor. The question alludes to the fact that, whenever possible, Rh-negative blood should be given to: Rh-negative patients who have either had a previous transfusion or may require a subsequent one, Rh-negative girls and women of childbearing age, mothers of infants who have haemolytic disease, or infants with haemolytic disease themselves. A Rh-positive patient can receive Rh-negative blood (125.1). A sound understanding of Rh incompatibility is important (125.2).

b) T In CPD and ACD 'D' is the abbreviation for dextrose. It is thought that dextrose provides energy for the synthesis of 2,3-DPG and adenosine triphosphate (125.2).

c) T Leucocyte depleted blood is indicated in patients with leucocyte antibodies who have experienced at least two febrile transfusion reactions (125.3).

d) T After 21 days storage whole blood may contain 30 mmol/l potassium (125.2).

e) F The recommended temperature for the storage of blood is 2–6°C. Blood that is transfused following freezing and thawing may cause death. However, blood may be stored at −79°C in glycerol and later rethawed for clinical use (125.2).

126a) T Standard bicarbonate is an indicator of the metabolic component of acid-base disturbance because it is a measure of acid-base status at normal P_{CO_2}. In metabolic alkalosis the bicarbonate is increased. Even if compensation takes place, the standard measurement will reveal the underlying metabolic component (126.1).

b) T With the occurrence of respiratory acidosis a metabolic compensation follows. Theoretically, in the early stages of a pure respiratory acidosis, standard bicarbonate may not change but the development of metabolic compensation will cause it to rise. Dangerous! (126.1).

c) F Standard bicarbonate illustrates the opposite, in other words the metabolic component. It is very easy to get mixed up here so be cautious (126.1).

d) T A working definition of standard bicarbonate is the concentration of bicarbonate ions per litre of plasma which has been equilibrated at 37°C with a gas mixture having P_{CO_2} 5.3 kPa (126.2).

e) F Standard base excess is a direct measure of the amount of strong acid required to bring the pH of the blood sample to 7.4 at P_{CO_2} 5.3 kPa at 37°C. Standard bicarbonate is, however, the concentration of bicarbonate ions in plasma that has been equilibrated to P_{CO_2} 5.3 kPa at 37°C. This measurement includes carbamino and CO_3^{3-} compounds in addition to HCO_3^- (126.1).

Also 15g Hb fully saturated

127 Fundamental biochemistry should be second nature. Difficulty with this question indicates a severe lack of preparation which needs to be remedied. <u>Do not guess.</u>

In comparing intracellular contents versus extracellular there is more:
a) phosphate
b) magnesium
c) ATP
d) chloride
e) sodium

128 Compliance is a concept which is well detailed in the standard texts on respiratory physiology. Remember that compliance and resistance are not interchangeable.

Compliance:
a) is greater in the neonate than adult
b) may be measured in vivo
c) is related to age
d) is related to lung volume
e) increases in consolidation

References

127.1 Harper	p 442
127.2 Guyton	p 20–21
128.1 Steward	p 13–14
128.2 West	p 156–157
128.3 Nunn	p 33–34

127a) T The intracellular phosphate concentration is 60 mmol/l whereas extracellular is 2 mmol/l (127.1).
 b) T The intracellular magnesium concentration is 30 mmol/l, extracellular 1.5 mmol/l (127.1).
 c) T ATP is exclusively an intracellular compound, 'a storehouse of energy' (127.2).
 d) F The chloride concentration is 100 mmol/l in the extracellular compartment whereas intracellular levels are extremely low (4 mmol/l) (127.1).
 e) F Sodium is the main extracellular cation at a concentration of 140 mmol/l whereas the intracellular concentration is much lower, 10 mmol/l (127.1).

128a) F At birth compliance is low but it increases slowly during the neonatal period and approximates to the adult value at 1 week (128.1).
 b) T Both static and dynamic compliance may be measured in vivo. The technique for doing so is documented in West (128.2).
 c) F There is surprisingly little change in compliance with age (but note that this excludes the first week of life). This is presumably due to the fact that lung elasticity is determined more by surface forces than tissue distensibility per se (128.3).
 d) T Compliance is directly related to lung volume. As Nunn so graphically states, 'an elephant has a much higher compliance than a mouse' (128.3).
 e) F Compliance, both specific and dynamic, is reduced in most forms of pulmonary pathology. These include collapse, consolidation, and fibrotic pleurisy (128.3). This should be obvious from clinical experience.

129 The physiology of the Valsalva manœuvre is ubiquitous. It may be asked in all three parts of the FRCAnaes. It is recommended that it is thoroughly known and understood.

The Valsalva manœuvre:
a) is forced expiration against a closed glottis
b) causes an initial increase in systemic blood pressure
c) causes bradycardia
d) reduces peripheral resistance
e) reduces preload

130 The physiological changes which occur on adopting a standing position from seated often partner the Valsalva manœuvre as a topic and are thus teamed together here.

In a fit adult, on standing from supine, arterial pressure:
a) rises in the carotid arteries
b) is unchanged in the legs
c) falls in cerebral arteries
d) falls in the thoracic aorta
e) falls leading to carotid body stimulation

References

129.1 Ganong	p 558–559
130.1 Ganong	p 583–584
130.2 Guyton	p 201

129a) T This is the definition of the Valsalva manœuvre (129.1).
  b) T Arterial pressure rises at the onset of straining due to the direct contribution of the sudden rise in intrathoracic pressure in aiding cardiac output. The effect is only temporary (129.1).
  c) F There is bradycardia on termination of the manœuvre due to the hypertension caused by restoring normal cardiac output into a constricted arterial tree (129.1).
  d) F The rise in peripheral resistance is secondary to the reduced cardiac output which is itself secondary to reduced venous return within the thorax (129.1).
  e) T True, after the initial phase of onset of straining when temporarily preload may be increased. See above (129.1).

130a) F Arterial pressure in the carotid arteries will fall due to simple gravitational effect (130.1).
  b) F Arterial pressure in the legs rises. This is due to gravitational influence (130.1).
  c) T In the same manner as for the carotid arteries, the arterial pressure in the cerebral vessels also falls due to gravitational effects (130.1).
  d) T This is true in general, although the precise change in arterial pressure relative to supine depends on the specific section of the thoracic aorta which is under consideration (130.1).
  e) T Although arterial pressure falls it is the baroreceptors which are stimulated. The carotid body has a chemoreceptor role but a drop in perfusion pressure which reduces carotid body blood flow will have a stimulant effect thereupon. Check with Question 55 if you are in any doubt (130.2).

131 The physiology of pregnancy encompasses several important haemo-dynamic features. The progressive changes which occur during pregnancy and their eventual resolution are a useful handle on which to peg viva questions. A specific revision text on obstetric anaesthesia will usually carry detail of the physiological changes in pregnancy.

In pregnancy:
a) cardiac output begins to increase during the 4th month
b) supine hypotensive syndrome may be present from the 28th week
c) plasma volume increases at term
d) serum albumin levels increase during the first 3 months
e) fibrinolytic activity is decreased

132 Despite the fact that the physiology of the gastrointestinal tract is of limited relevance to anaesthetic practice, the wealth of material that it encapsulates provides ample scope for discussion.

Pancreatic juice contains:
a) chymotrypsin
b) trypsin
c) enterolipase
d) enterokinase
e) amylase

References
131.1 Datta   p 3
131.2 Datta   p 152–153
131.3 Moir   p 9–10
131.4 Moir   p 12
131.5 Moir   p 14–15

132.1 Guyton   p 718–719

131a) F It is fair to say that there is a degree of uncertainty in respect of the cardiovascular changes which occur during pregnancy but certain views are generally held. One of these is that cardiac output rises considerably during the first trimester. The response to this completion is therefore 'false' (131.1).
  b) T Supine hypotensive syndrome is well recognized in gravida (131.2). It is generally not seen before the 28th week unless polyhydramnios or multiple pregnancy are contributory factors.
  c) F The plasma volume increases from the 6th week of pregnancy until about 34 weeks, after which it remains fairly constant (131.3).
  d) F Plasma albumin falls by 10 g/l but plasma globulins and fibrinogen are actually increased (131.4).
  e) T Fibrinolytic activity is reduced and fibrinogen levels are higher (131.5).

132a) T Chymotrypsin is one of the proteolytic enzymes secreted by the pancreas (132.1).
  b) T Trypsin is secreted by the pancreas. In order to prevent self-digestion, trypsin inhibitor is secreted concomitantly. This is stored in the cytoplasm of the glandular cells and prevents the trypsin acting within the acini and ducts of the pancreas (132.1).
  c) T Pancreatic lipase is one of the main enzymes involved in fat digestion (132.1).
  d) T Enterokinase is responsible for the activation of trypsinogen and is secreted when chyme comes into contact with the mucosa (132.1).
  e) T Amylase is present in pancreatic juice. Its role is that of hydrolysing starches and glycogen (132.1).

133 With respect to the physiology of clotting it is all too easy to become confused between the numerical factors and their various roles. It will pay to have a clear mnemonic or other tool to aid recollection. Make sure you can sketch the clotting cascade.

The following are common to both intrinsic and extrinsic clotting pathways:
a) factor VII
b) factor V
c) factor VIII
d) factor IX
e) calcium

134 While the question above is very much a test of memory this one is more concerned with the understanding of the actual physiology underlying the mechanism of clotting.

With respect to the mechanism of clotting:
a) thrombin is a catalyst for the conversion of fibrinogen to fibrin.
b) tissue thromboplastin triggers the intrinsic system
c) heparin is a cofactor for antithrombin III
d) activated factor IX causes the conversion of prothrombin to thrombin
e) factor X is activated by both intrinsic and extrinsic systems

References

133.1 Guyton	p 393–395
133.2 Ganong	p 500
134.1 Ganong	p 499–503
134.2 Guyton	p 393–395

133a) F Factor VII (serum prothrombin conversion accelerator) features in the extrinsic system only (133.1).
  b) T Factor V (proaccelerin or labile factor) is common to both extrinsic and intrinsic pathways (133.2).
  c) F Factor VIII (antihaemophilic factor) is featured in the intrinsic pathway. Its role is to act in concert with factor IX (Christmas factor) to activate factor X (133.1).
  d) F Factor IX (plasma thromboplastin component) occurs in the intrinsic pathway. It acts together with factor VIII (133.2).
  e) T Calcium ions have a role in both pathways (133.2).

134a) T The conversion of fibrinogen to fibrin is catalysed by thrombin, a serum protease which itself is formed from prothrombin (134.2).
  b) F It is the extrinsic system which is triggered by the local release of tissue thromboplastin (134.1).
  c) T Antithrombin III is a circulating protease inhibitor that binds to the serine proteases in the clotting cascade and prevents their clotting activity. Heparin, acting as a cofactor, facilitates this binding (134.1).
  d) F It is factor X that catalyses this process but the conversion of prothrombin to thrombin is actually caused by prothrombin activator (134.2).
  e) T Factor X may be activated by both pathways (134.2).

135 Neurophysiology can easily become the Cinderella of revision. It is wise to be informed about the pathways in the nervous system and functions of the cerebellum and basal ganglia. Within this field formation and drainage of CSF is a frequent topic. See Questions 136 and 44.

The following regulate hypothalamic function:
a) sleep
b) appetite
c) fear
d) sexual arousal
e) limbic pathways

136 Cerebrospinal fluid has several roles. The most important of these is the cushioning of the brain within its solid vault. A minor nutritional role has been suggested but is unproven.

Cerebrospinal fluid:
a) is formed at 200 ml/h
b) has the same composition as brain ECF
c) contains urea
d) is iso-osmotic with plasma
e) drains into the canal of Schlemm

References	
135.1 Ganong	p 215–217
135.2 Ganong	p 218–222
136.1 Ganong	p 563
136.2 Ganong	p 564
136.3 Ganong	p 136

135a) F There is a variety of opinion concerning the role of the hypo-thalamus in the regulation of sleep patterns. There is a great deal of controversy surrounding the existence of 'sleep' and 'wake' centres and the hypothalamus is not indisputably connected with sleep patterns. It seems unlikely that sleep patterns have any unique or direct role in the regulation of hypothalamic function (135.1).

b) T In contrast to the above there is an intimate connection between hypothalamic function and appetite and satiety (135.2). There is an interaction between the feeding centre and satiety centre which has relevance to the syndrome of hypothalamic obesity characterized by hyperphagia.

c) T Defensive reactions, fear and rage affect the function of the hypothalamus and incorporate input from the limbic system (135.1).

d) T The mechanism is mediated by cells which are sensitive to circulating hormones such as oestrogens and androgens (135.1).

e) T The limbic system is the integrating system for the regulatory role of the fear and rage effects referred to above (135.1).

136a) F This value is far too high. The correct figure for CSF formation is in the region of 500 ml/24 h (136.1).

b) T The composition of CSF is exactly the same as that of brain extracellular fluid (136.1). It should, however, be noted that CSF is most certainly not identical in composition with plasma — a frequently posed question.

c) T Urea is present in CSF at an approximate concentration of 120 mg/l (136.2).

d) T CSF has an identical osmolality to plasma. This is 290 mosmol/kg H_2O (136.2). Note the comments above on ionic composition.

e) F CSF circulates via the foramina of Magendie and Luscka. The canal of Schlemm is in the eye (136.1) (136.3). This is obviously a deliberate attempt to mislead. It will always catch out a few candidates, so take your time to think!

137 In the College of Anaesthetists' guide to the examination it is notable that the importance of cardiovascular physiology along with respiratory and neurophysiology is deliberately emphasized. You are advised to read this document. The following two questions concentrate on the cardiovascular system.

Pulse pressure is lowest in the:
a) aorta
b) femoral artery
c) dorsalis pedis artery
d) arterioles
e) capillaries

138 Once again it must be stressed that there should be no confusion in your mind as to the precise roles of the carotid body and carotid sinus.

A rise in blood pressure in the carotid sinus will cause:
a) a reduction in vagal tone
b) reduced sympathetic discharge to the heart
c) increased vasomotor activity
d) increased heart rate
e) a fall in mean arterial pressure

References	
137.1 Ganong	p 541–542
137.2 Ganong	p 545–546
138.1 Ganong	p 555–556
138.2 Scurr, Feldman & Soni	p 161–163
138.3 Guyton	p 198–201

137a) F Pulse pressure may be defined as the difference between the systolic and diastolic pressure within the vessel and is normally about 50 mmHg in large vessels. The pulse pressure falls very slightly in large and medium sized vessels because their resistance to flow is small but it falls very rapidly in the small vessels. Pulse pressure declines rapidly in arterioles to about 5 mmHg at their distal ends (137.1).

b) F The pulse pressure in the femoral artery will be less than in the aorta for the reasons above but still greater than in smaller vessels (137.1).

c) F Exactly the same logic applies here (137.1). The wording of the stem is not the best possible as it appears to imply that only one completion is true. On this occasion that is actually the case but such questions are uncommon.

d) F From the above information this might appear to be true but capillaries have a pulse pressure of their own which is approximately 5 mmHg at the arteriolar end and zero at the venous end (137.2).

e) T The 5 mmHg pulse pressure in capillaries is the lowest (137.2).

138a) F The carotid sinus contains baroreceptors, the afferent fibres of which combine with the fibres from the carotid body and form the carotid sinus nerve. The carotid sinus nerve is a branch of the glossopharyngeal nerve (ninth cranial). When the pressure in the carotid sinus rises the discharge rate increases, and correspondingly when the pressure falls the rate declines (138.1).

b) T High pressure mechanoreceptors such as the carotid sinus are attenuated by lower blood pressures. Heart rate and inotropy are augmented by an increase in cardiac sympathetic tone when the pressure within mechanoreceptors falls. The reverse sequence also occurs hence the answer to this completion is 'true' (138.2).

c) F Vasomotor activity is reduced and vasodilatation occurs (138.3). There is a fall in cardiac output and a decrease in heart rate arising from medullary effects.

d) F Heart rate falls due to vagal stimulation (138.3). This arises from stimulation of the vagal centre in the medulla.

e) T The mean arterial pressure falls. This response is limited to the range 30–150 mmHg (138.1).

139 The properties of hormones which may be asked include their physiological actions, site and method of production, and regulation of secretion. In MCQ format questions based on hormones can be alarmingly wide ranging. Glucagon is one of the more familiar hormones.

Glucagon:
a) activates phosphorylase kinase
b) inhibits gluconeogenesis
c) causes glycogenolysis
d) activates muscle phosphorylase
e) secretion is inhibited by somatostatin

140 Aldosterone is responsible for most of the mineralocorticoid activity of the adrenal cortex. It occupies a central position in volume homeostasis and is intimately concerned with the metabolic response to surgery and trauma. Compare Question 65.

Aldosterone secretion is stimulated by:
a) potassium
b) renin
c) ACTH
d) a reduction in sodium intake
e) surgery

References
139.1 Guyton   p 862–863
139.2 Guyton   p 752
139.3 Ganong   p 326–327
139.4 Guyton   p 747
139.5 Guyton   p 863

140.1 Guyton   p 845–846
140.2 Ganong   p 355–357

139a) T Glucagon has two major effects on glucose metabolism: breakdown of liver glycogen (glycogenolysis); and increased production of glucose from amino acids and the glycerol portion of fat (gluconeogenesis) (139.1) (139.2). Glucagon causes glycogenolysis within the liver which in turn increases blood glucose concentration within minutes. There is a complex cascade of events as follows: glucagon activates adenyl cyclase in the hepatic cell membrane and this causes formation of cyclic AMP which activates protein kinase regulator protein which in turn activates protein kinase. This activates phosphorylase b kinase which converts phosphorylase b into phosphorylase a which promotes the degradation of glycogen into glucose-1-phosphate which is then dephosphorylated to form glucose which is released from the liver cells (139.2).

b) F Glucagon is gluconeogenic even after the exhaustion of liver glycogen, by an effect on liver cells. The precise mechanism is not known (139.2).

c) T Glucagon is glycogenolytic. Glycogenolysis is the breakdown of glycogen (139.2).

d) F Glucagon does not cause glycogenolysis in muscle (139.3). Phosphorylase can be activated by both adrenaline and glucagon. Adrenaline activates phosphorylase via cyclic AMP in both liver and muscle but glucagon activates phosphorylase 'mainly' in the liver (139.4).

e) T Somatostatin has many functions including the elevation of blood glucose. There are also multiple inhibitory effects as follows: there is local depression of insulin and glucagon secretion from the islets of Langerhans; motility of stomach duodenum and the gallbladder is decreased; and somatostatin decreases both secretion and absorption in the gastrointestinal tract (139.5).

140a) T An increase in potassium ion concentration of less than 1 mmol/l will triple the rate of aldosterone secretion (140.1). There are four different factors presently known to play essential roles in the regulation of aldosterone secretion. In order of importance these are: potassium ion concentration of the extracellular fluid; the renin–angiotensin system; the quantity of body sodium; and adrenocorticotrophic hormone (ACTH).

b) T Aldosterone secretion is regulated via the renin–angiotensin system in a feedback loop. A fall in ECF volume or intra-arterial vascular volume leads to a reflex increase in renal nerve discharge and a decrease in renal arterial pressure. Both these changes increase renin secretion. Angiotensin II formed by the action of the renin increases the rate of secretion of aldosterone (140.2).

c) T ACTH is the anterior pituitary hormone that controls the secretion of glucocorticoids. ACTH also has a permissive effect on aldosterone. All other forms of regulation of secretion of aldosterone will only occur if there is a minimal amount of ACTH present (140.1).

d) T After several days of sodium deficient diet the rate of aldosterone secretion increases despite there being no change in sodium ion concentration of the body fluids. (140.1).

e) T Factors which increase secretion of aldosterone include surgery, anxiety, physical trauma, and haemorrhage (140.1).

141 REM sleep has a very different EEG pattern to other activities including the anaesthetised state. Refer to Question 69.

The condition known as REM sleep:
a) is that point at which the individual becomes aware and alert
b) is characterized by slow, high voltage regular EEG activity
c) is referred to as paradoxical sleep
d) causes inhibition of peripheral muscles
e) increases growth hormone production

142 The physiological role of carbon dioxide is closely related to metabolism at a cellular level. Frequently carriage and excretion of CO_2 will be met in the examination. The question below refers to exogenous carbon dioxide, a different approach.

Breathing CO_2 for prolonged periods will result in:
a) only alveolar P_{CO_2} rising
b) only tissue P_{CO_2} decreasing
c) alveolar ventilation decreasing
d) both alveolar and tissue P_{CO_2} increasing
e) liver cirrhosis

References	
141.1 Guyton	p 659–660
141.2 Ganong	p 381
142.1 Nunn	p 226–228
142.2 Nunn	p 224
142.3 Nunn	p 219
142.4 Nunn	p 460–470
142.5 Atkinson, Rushman & Lee	p 343

141a) F This is false although people do usually wake in the morning from REM sleep rather than from slow wave sleep. During REM sleep people are more difficult to arouse by sensory stimuli (141.1).

b) F Slow, high voltage, regular EEG activity is a characteristic of slow wave sleep. In REM sleep the EEG generally shows a de-synchronized pattern of beta waves similar to those seen in an awake state. REM sleep is sometimes called paradoxical sleep because it is a paradox that a person can still be asleep despite marked activity in the brain on the EEG (141.1).

c) T Exactly as detailed above. The paradox is the presence of such a high level of cerebral electrical activity in a sleeping state (141.1).

d) T Muscle tone throughout the body is exceedingly depressed which indicates strong inhibition of spinal projections from the reticular formation of the brain stem. Despite this inhibition, a few irregular muscle movements occur including rapid eye movements, hence the name REM sleep (141.1).

e) F Growth hormone secretion is increased in subjects deprived of REM sleep. Secretion of growth hormone is inhibited during REM sleep (141.2). The precise significance of this is not understood.

142a) F There really is an alveolar/arterial P_{CO_2} gradient. Because of the small difference there is an established convention by which the arterial and alveolar P_{CO_2} values are taken to be identical. It is obvious that arterial P_{CO_2} will rise along with alveolar P_{CO_2} in the absence of a diffusion barrier (142.1).

b) F All membranes permit the rapid diffusion of carbon dioxide. Therefore if arterial P_{CO_2} rises then tissue P_{CO_2} will rise also (142.2) (142.3).

c) F There is a linear relationship between Pa_{CO_2} and alveolar ventilation until approximately 10.7 kPa. As Pa_{CO_2} rises above this level a point of maximal ventilatory stimulation is reached (between 13.3 and 26.7 kPa). Thereafter ventilatory stimulation is reduced until apnoea occurs (142.3).

d) T This is a combination of the answers to a) and b) above (142.1) (142.2).

e) F Beware! A chapter on 'The effects of changes in carbon dioxide tension' makes no references to liver damage of any kind (142.4). However, a different source states 'hypercapnia is a factor in producing liver damage' (142.5).

143 The systemic and pulmonary circulations differ in function and structure. Knowledge of the mechanics of each and the values for flow and pressure is essential to answer this question.

In contrast to the systemic circulation, the pulmonary circulation is characterized by:
a) a lower mean pressure
b) a higher resistance
c) a relatively small pulse pressure
d) a larger volume flow per minute
e) the absence of sympathetic control

144 Renal physiology is closely related to homeostasis. Glucose is handled by the kidney in a unique way and it shares a carrier mechanism with sodium. Draw a distinction between active and passive reabsorption.

Active reabsorption of glucose occurs in the:
a) proximal tubules
b) loops of Henle
c) distal tubules
d) collecting ducts
e) bladder

References

143.1 West	p 32
143.2 West	p 35
143.3 Ganong	p 611–612
143.4 Nunn	p 117
143.5 Nunn	p 126–127
144.1 Ganong	p 660–661
144.2 Lote	p 58–62
144.3 Guyton	p 302–305

143a) T In the pulmonary circulation the arterial pressure and vascular resistance are approximately one sixth of those found in the systemic circulation. The mean pressure in the pulmonary artery is 15 mmHg (25/8) and in systemic arteries is 100 mmHg (120/80) (143.1). The figures in brackets are systolic and diastolic values.

b) F The pulmonary vascular resistance is very low, about 1.7 mmHg/l min^{-1} or 100 dynes.s.cm^{-5} (143.2).

c) T The pulse pressure is defined as the difference between systolic and diastolic pressures. For typical values the pulse pressure in the systemic circulation is 40 mmHg and that in the pulmonary circulation 15 mmHg (143.3).

d) F The flow of blood through the pulmonary circulation is approximately equal to that through the systemic circulation. The figure for this varies between 6 l/min and about 25 l/min (143.4).

e) F The pulmonary circulation is under both sympathetic and, to a lesser degree, parasympathetic control (143.5).

144a) T Glucose is reabsorbed in the early part of the proximal convoluted tubule (PCT) together with amino acids, bicarbonate, and sodium. The mechanism of glucose reabsorption in the kidney is based on a common carrier for both glucose and sodium in the luminal membrane. Glucose is subsequently carried into the cell as sodium follows its concentration gradient. This is a process of secondary active transport (144.1).

b) F The mechanism of active reabsorption for glucose may function further along the nephron than the early part of the PCT (144.2). Despite this, however, there is no glucose remaining in the fluid entering the loop of Henle. Thus distal to the PCT there is no active reabsorption (144.3).

c) F By the same reasoning as above there is no active reabsorption of glucose in the distal tubule (144.3).

d) F There is no active reabsorption of glucose in the collecting ducts (144.3).

e) F The bladder acts as a storage organ only. The above statements also apply (144.3).

145 The physiological effects of extreme altitude or depth on the internal milieu comprise a topic which incorporates important principles of direct relevance to anaesthesia. Some knowledge of basic physics will help here. Divers and climbers should enjoy these two questions.

In acclimatization to altitude:
a) initially hyperventilation occurs
b) the oxygen haemoglobin dissociation curve shifts to the right
c) erythropoietin secretion increases
d) tissue content of cytochrome oxidase is increased
e) P_{50} is increased

146 The physiological responses to depth are not simply the opposite of those seen in acclimatization to altitude. Consider carefully before you attempt this question.

With regard to increased atmospheric pressure:
a) gas density increases in direct proportion to pressure
b) maximal breathing capacity is reduced
c) inspired P_{O_2} increases along with pressure
d) nitrogen may have a profound anaesthetic effect at depth
e) the solubility of nitrogen in blood is reduced

References	
145.1 Ganong	p 637–638
146.1 Nunn	p 324–325

145a) T Initially in acclimatization there may be a transient 'mountain sickness' phase which has hyperventilation as one of its features (145.1).

b) T The hyperventilation shifts the oxygen haemoglobin dissociation curve to the left as the alkalosis develops. There is also an elevation of red cell 2,3-DPG which tends to decrease the oxygen affinity of haemoglobin. The net result is an increase in P_{50} (145.1).

c) T Erythropoietin secretion promptly increases on ascent to high altitude (145.1).

d) T Other compensatory changes occur as well as the shift in the curve. Among the more important of these is the increase in myoglobin and tissue cytochrome oxidase (145.1).

e) T This is the net result of the shift in the oxygen haemoglobin dissociation curve and the increase in red cell 2,3-DPG which accompanies it (145.1).

146a) T Gas density increases in direct proportion to increasing pressure. Air at 5 atmospheres (atm) has five times the density of air at sea level (146.1).

b) T To some extent this is a corollary of a). Maximal breathing capacity (MBC) is reduced due to the extra work of breathing engendered by the higher density of gas. In respect of air, MBC may be reduced by half at 5 atm ambient pressure (146.1).

c) T True, although it is notable that the proportional change is greater than that of pressure alone. This is due to the saturated vapour pressure of water being unchanged (146.1).

d) T Nitrogen is an anaesthetic agent and may cause full surgical anaesthesia at 30 atm. Even at 4 atm there is a clinical narcotic effect (146.1).

e) F Nitrogen becomes increasingly soluble at depth. While there is no problem in this state of affairs during compression, decompression will cause bubbles of nitrogen to evolve in the tissues leading to the syndrome known as the 'bends' which is characterized by joint pains, itching, paralysis, and dyspnoea (146.1).

147 The thyroid gland is not the only subject under scrutiny in this question. One of the strengths of MCQ papers from the examiners' point of view is their ability to cover a lot of ground in a single question.

The following are true of thyroid hormones:
a) triiodothyronine occurs in a reverse form
b) thyroxine is a prohormone
c) they increase nitrogen excretion
d) in pregnancy thyroxine binding globulin is reduced
e) long acting thyroid stimulating hormone is secreted by the thyroid gland

148 Basal metabolic rate (BMR) has its own rigid definition which is necessary to answer this question. Nutritional topics related to BMR may also occur in the examination.

Basal metabolic rate:
a) is 3000 kcal/24 h for a 70 kg man
b) is increased by anxiety
c) is increased by 20% for each °C rise in temperature
d) falls in starvation
e) is higher in the tropics

References	
147.1 Harper	p 487
147.2 Ganong	p 302
147.3 Ganong	p 303
147.4 Ganong	p 301
147.5 Ganong	p 307
148.1 Ganong	p 236–264

147a) T Normal triiodothyronine is 3,5,3-triiodothyronine but the reverse form 3,3,5-triiodothyronine is also produced by the gland (147.1).

b) T There is some room for debate over the status of thyroxine as a prohormone. It is believed that T_4 (thyroxine) is inert until converted to T_3. While it is difficult to prove that T_4 has no activity of its own the fact that it is the major precursor of T_3 qualifies it as a prohormone (147.2).

c) T The thyroid hormones all increase metabolic rate and catabolism. Hence nitrogen excretion is increased (147.3).

d) F The level of thyroid binding globulin is increased in pregnancy (147.4).

e) F LATS has been shown to be an immunoglobulin (not a hormone) which causes thyroid stimulation. These immunoglobulins are produced by circulating plasma cells, not the gland itself (147.5).

148a) F The correct figure is much lower at around 2000 kcal/24 h (148.1). Basal metabolic rate (BMR) is measured at rest in a room of comfortable temperature 12 h after a meal.

b) T Emotional state has a direct effect on metabolic rate. BMR is elevated by anxiety (148.1).

c) F BMR is increased by 14% or so for each °C rise in body temperature (148.1).

d) T During prolonged starvation BMR paradoxically falls (148.1).

e) T Although BMR is defined as the metabolic rate at rest 12 h after a meal in a room of constant temperature, it is nevertheless higher in warmer climates (148.1).

149 Even the simplest questions on the oxygen haemoglobin dissociation curve can cause confusion. On first sight of the question sketch the curve and its changes on the question paper. It will then be possible to work from the sketch logically.

The oxygen haemoglobin dissociation curve:
a) is shifted to the left in pulmonary capillaries
b) is shifted to the left in hypothermia
c) is shifted to the left in acidaemia
d) is shifted to the left on replacing HbA by HbF_2
e) shifts to the left to increase oxygen availability

150 Transferrin has an important physiological role in the transport of iron. While transferrin may not appear an obvious revision topic, it is nonetheless featured in the examination at regular intervals. Do not confuse transferrin with apotransferritin for the two have differing parts to play in iron transfer and storage.

Transferrin:
a) is involved in the transfer of ferrous ions to the gastric cells
b) circulates in the plasma
c) is involved in the transfer of iron to the liver
d) is involved in the transfer of iron to red cells
e) delivers iron to the mitochondria

References	
149.1 Guyton	p 438
149.2 Nunn	p 258–73
150.1 Guyton	p 361–362
150.2 Ganong	p 446–447

149a) T As blood passes through the pulmonary capillaries, carbon dioxide diffuses from it, reducing the carbonic acid content and decreasing hydrogen ion concentration. These effects shift the oxygen haemoglobin dissociation curve to the left and upwards. This is the Bohr effect (149.1).

b) T The curve shifts to the left with a fall in body temperature (149.1). In general, factors that are reduced, such as temperature, will cause a left shift whilst an increase causes a right shift.

c) F When blood pH falls to 7.2 the curve shifts on average 15% to the right (149.1). The apparent paradox of a <u>decrease</u> in pH causing a <u>right</u> shift is eliminated if a rise in pH is considered as a reduction in hydrogen ion concentration.

d) T HbF_2 is fetal haemoglobin. The curve moves to the left in the presence of large quantities of fetal haemoglobin (149.1).

e) F A shift to the left of the curve implies a decrease in available oxygen to the tissues (149.2).

150a) T Ferrous ions (Fe^{2+}) are absorbed from the small intestine after which they combine with the beta globulin apotransferritin to form transferrin which circulates in the plasma. The binding is loose and iron may be released to any cells at any part of the circulation (150.1).

b) T Transferrin is a polypeptide which freely circulates in the plasma (150.2).

c) T As detailed above. The liver is the major site of the deposition of iron (150.2).

d) T Transferrin has a unique feature of binding to receptors on the cell membranes of erythroblasts. It is subsequently ingested into the cell by a process of endocytosis. The iron is then delivered directly to the mitochondria for haem synthesis (150.1).

e) T Direct delivery of iron to the mitochondria occurs (150.1).

151 Knowledge of the physiology of cardiac function is vital. It is mandatory for the safe practice of anaesthesia and has important applications in the understanding of pre-existing disease states.

Myocardial contractility:
a) may be defined as a change in force of contraction at any given fibre length
b) is affected by preload
c) is inhibited by an increase in intracellular calcium
d) depends on Starling's law
e) is affected by heart rate

152 It is useful to be able to reproduce the determinants of cardiac output in tabular form. If you do not already have a revision table, suitable sources will be found in the references below.

The following are determinants of cardiac output:
a) heart rate
b) stroke volume
c) preload
d) afterload
e) sympathetic stimulation

References	
151.1 Ganong	p 529–530
151.2 Ganong	p 528
152.1 Ganong	p 527–528
152.2 Ganong	p 530

151a) T This is quite a rigid definition and as it stands would exclude the effects of varying left ventricular end diastolic volume. If the phrase 'at any given fibre length' is omitted then a more universal definition results (151.1).

b) T This is true in as much as the volume–contraction relationship applies (Starling's law). If the more rigid definition above is applied then factors which alter fibre length per se will not be included (151.1).

c) F Myocardial contractility is enhanced when the availability of intracellular calcium is increased (151.1).

d) T Starling's law states that 'energy of contraction is proportional to the initial length of the cardiac muscle fibre' (151.2).

e) T Myocardial contractility increases as heart rate increases although this effect is not great (151.1).

152a) T Cardiac output may be defined as stroke volume multiplied by heart rate (152.1).

b) T This should be obvious from the above definition of cardiac output (152.1). It is very fundamental physiology.

c) T An increase in the ventricular filling volume caused by preload alters cardiac output in the manner described above by Starling's law (152.1).

d) T After an increase in afterload, or the resistance to flow from the aortic valve, as it may be put, the heart pumps out less blood than it receives for several beats. Later reflex mechanisms come into play to limit the effect (152.1).

e) T Sympathetic stimulation has a direct effect which increases myocardial contractility (152.2).

153 The field of acid-base balance is fraught with pitfalls for the trainee, most of which are due to poor understanding of the subject. In particular the interpretation of the results of blood gas analysis with respect to the quantification of respiratory and metabolic components of a disturbance can be difficult. Try to think through the situation logically before attempting the question. Avoid ambiguous completions.

Respiratory alkalosis is seen in:
a) sleep
b) hysteria
c) hyperventilation
d) metabolic acidosis
e) metabolic alkalosis

154 Although the commonest questions on blood and transfusion are based on compatibility reactions remember that there are other possibilities. This example is based on the composition of blood.

Compared with fresh whole blood, stored blood has:
a) more platelets
b) more 2,3-DPG
c) increased extracellular potassium
d) increased extracellular haemoglobin
e) increased factor VIII

References

153.1 Nunn	p 304
153.2 Ganong	p 642–643
153.3 Guyton	p 340–341
154.1 Atkinson, Rushman & Lee	p 818
154.2 Mollinson	p 136–138
154.3 Miller	p 1473

153a) F Arterial Pco_2 is usually slightly elevated during sleep (about 0.4 kPa) (153.1). If there is any change in blood pH there will be a respiratory acidosis.

b) T Provided that the hysteria is associated with hyperventilation (which may not always be the case) then hypocapnia will occur and a respiratory alkalosis of pH 7.5 to 7.6 will be an accompaniment (153.2).

c) T Hyperventilation produces hypocapnia with associated respiratory alkalosis (153.2).

d) T In metabolic acidosis the plasma hydrogen ion concentration rises and pulmonary ventilation increases to compensate. Rapid removal of carbon dioxide occurs and the hydrogen ion concentration moves back towards normal. This compensation is only partial (50–75%) but a compensatory respiratory alkalosis of some degree will usually be seen (153.3).

e) F A metabolic alkalosis diminishes the pulmonary ventilation which in turn increases hydrogen ion concentration. Again compensation of 50–75% or so will occur but there is no reason why respiratory alkalosis should be seen (153.3).

154a) F CPD blood (citrate-phosphate-dextrose) contains very few functioning platelets (154.1).

b) F 2, 3-DPG levels fall progressively with time of storage (154.2). CPD blood suffers less in this regard than does ACD blood.

c) T Extracellular potassium concentration in stored blood is raised and may reach 30 mmol/l or so after 30–35 days storage (154.2).

d) T This is true although the rate of haemolysis is low (for example in ACD blood fewer than 1% of cells have haemolysed after 42 days) (154.2).

e) F Factor VIII is reduced to 10% of its original level after 1 week's storage of CPD blood. Today most blood contains SAGM storage medium (saline-adenine-glucose-mannitol) from which plasma and clotting factors have been removed (154.1).

155 Angiotensin I and II and the physiology of the conversion process thereof form an area of current interest. This field is open to change as it is an area of rapidly advancing knowledge. Remember angiotensin III also.

The following statements are true of angiotensin II:
a) it stimulates renin release
b) it is released by the adrenal medulla
c) it acts on vascular smooth muscle
d) it is formed in the lung
e) it is secreted in response to hyponatraemia

156 Renin has intimate connections with the angiotensin system. It has a profound role itself in the maintenance of circulating volume.

Renin secretion is increased by the following:
a) haemorrhage
b) dehydration
c) upright posture
d) cirrhosis of the liver
e) hypotension

References	
155.1 Ganong	p 426–428
156.1 Ganong	p 428–430

155a) F Angiotensin II, a potent vasoconstrictor, feeds back on to the renin release mechanism to inhibit it (155.1). This effect is mediated by a direct action on juxtaglomerular cells. Angiotensin III has less pressor activity but strangely just as much aldosterone stimulating effect.

b) F Angiotensin II is formed from angiotensin I in the plasma by the cleavage of ACE (angiotensin converting enzyme). It is not formed in the adrenal gland (155.1).

c) T Angiotensin II, one of the most potent vasoconstrictiors known, is about five times more potent than noradrenaline (155.1). Note the comment above on angiotensin III.

d) T The lung is the major site for conversion of angiotensin I to angiotensin II (155.1).

e) T In hyponatraemic states the pressor response to angiotensin II is reduced and circulating levels of angiotensin II become elevated (155.1).

156a) T Renin secretion is increased by factors which decrease ECF volume; one of them is obviously haemorrhage (156.1).

b) T The mechanism is identical to the above (156.1).

c) T There is an intrarenal baroreceptor response which causes renin secretion to increase when intra-arteriolar pressure in the juxtaglomerular apparatus is reduced (156.1).

d) T Although the reason for this effect in cirrhosis is not precisely clear (156.1).

e) T Hypotension has the same effect as a reduction in the ECF volume (156.1).

157 The weighting of the examination in favour of cardiac, respiratory, and neurophysiology has been alluded to previously. Spinal cord transection can provide illumination on the transmission of information within the spinal cord as the following questions show.

In complete cord transection:
a) hyperreflexia occurs initially
b) arterial blood pressure will not change
c) new nerve endings may sprout in the cord
d) the stretch reflex is the first to return
e) bladder control remains throughout

158 The terminology used to describe spinal cord transection is variable. The question below is based on identical physiology to the one above although the wording may obscure this fact.

The following statements are true of spinal shock:
a) all spinal reflex responses are depressed
b) in humans the phase lasts one week
c) denervation hypersensitivity develops
d) the resting membrane potential of spinal motor neurones is increased by 5 mV
e) in the recovery phase hyperreflexia is seen

References	
157.1 Guyton	p 601
158.1 Ganong	p 193–195

157a) F All spinal cord functions, including cord reflexes, immediately become profoundly depressed after spinal cord transection to a state of 'oblivion' or spinal shock. This situation may last for days or weeks in humans (157.1). Hyperreflexia is seen at a later stage.

b) F Blood pressure will fall immediately to as low as 40 mmHg due to complete blockade of sympathetic activity (157.1).

c) T The sprouting of multiple new nerve endings in the cord may contribute to the increase in reflex excitability which develops later (157.1).

d) T The stretch reflex is the first to return, followed by progressively more complex reflexes in sequence (157.1). *bulbocavernous + anal reflex*

e) F The sacral reflexes that control bladder and colon evacuation are completely suppressed for the first few weeks (157.1).

158a) T The spinal shock that follows transection of the cord is characterized by profound depression of spinal reflex response (158.1). This is detailed above.

b) F The duration of spinal shock is variable but it is usually for a period of 2 weeks minimum (158.1).

c) T The recovery of reflex excitability results from the development of denervation hypersensitivity (158.1). A contributory mechanism is the sprouting of new nerve endings (157.1).

d) T The resting membrane potential of the spinal motor neurones is 2–6 mV higher than normal (158.1).

e) T Initially all reflexes are profoundly depressed. In contrast during the recovery phase of spinal shock reflexes not only return but also become hyperactive (158.1).

159 The last two questions of this physiology batch relate to the circulation through special regions. Cerebral blood flow is vital to the organism. It follows that a degree of inbuilt regulation will exist to protect the brain against hypoxia. That is so but other mechanisms are also important.

Cerebral blood flow:
a) is equally divided between internal carotid and vertebral arteries
b) shows large regional variations
c) is equal to cardiac output
d) is susceptible to changes in arterial P_{CO_2}
e) is affected by local mediators

160 Coronary blood flow has different determinants than those of cerebral blood flow but some factors are common to both. The anatomy of the coronary circulation will prove helpful.

Coronary artery blood flow:
a) has diastolic blood pressure as the major determinant
b) is unaffected by changes in mean arterial pressure
c) is mainly under humoral control
d) increases in response to hypoxia
e) receives 85% of venous return via the coronary sinus

References

159.1 Ganong	p 562
159.2 Ganong	p 568–569
159.3 Guyton	p 679–681
160.1 Scurr, Feldman & Soni	p 183
160.2 Ganong	p 573–576

159a) F In humans most cerebral blood flow is supplied by the carotid arteries with only a small fraction contributed by the vertebral arteries (159.1).

b) T There are large fluctuations in regional blood flow dependent on area and type of activity in each area. A gross example is seen in the grey matter where blood flow is about six times that in white matter (159.2). Another example is seen in the motor cortex where the relevant area of involvement with a particular motor group will show an increase in local blood flow when that motor group is in action.

c) F The average cerebral blood flow in young adults is 50–55 ml/100 g min^{-1} or 750 ml/min, approximately 15% of the total resting cardiac output (159.3).

d) T Cerebral blood flow is proportional to both arterial and venous P_{CO_2} subject to an upper and lower limit. A graphic representation is useful (159.3).

e) T Locally released mediators (such as metabolic products) have a direct effect in their own vicinity (159.2). Circulating peptides such as angiotensin II will also have an effect.

160a) T Coronary artery flow increases rapidly in diastole and then decreases linearly as diastolic pressure falls and the intracavitary pressure of the left ventricle rises (160.1).

b) F There is an autoregulatory range where steady state flow rate is relatively independent of perfusion pressure. This range extends between 60 and 120 mmHg. Outside this range perfusion becomes linearly related to pressure (160.1).

c) F Coronary artery flow is influenced largely by autoregulation (160.2). Humoral factors may have a role, for example noradrenaline will cause coronary vasoconstriction but this will always be overcome by hypoxia.

d) T Hypoxia increases blood flow by 200–300% in denervated and intact hearts (160.2).

e) F Of the total coronary blood flow 75% drains from left ventricular muscle by way of the coronary sinus. Most of the venous blood from right ventricular muscle flows through the anterior cardiac veins directly into the right atrium. A small amount of coronary blood flows back into the heart through thebesian veins which empty directly into all chambers of the heart (160.2).

161 At first it looks as though this topic belongs more under physiology than pharmacology. A closer look will reveal that the nub of the question is the effects of various drugs on the pulmonary vasculature. Some completions may be deduced from first principles.

Reflex pulmonary vasoconstriction is abolished by:
a) oxygen
b) tolazoline
c) adrenaline
d) almitrine
e) carbon dioxide

162 The inhibitors of monoamine oxidase appear more often in this examination than in clinical practice (thankfully for anaesthetists). Only respond to those completions of which you are sure.

Patients receiving monoamine oxidase inhibitors may react adversely to:
a) butter
b) cheese
c) noradrenaline
d) amphetamines
e) chianti

References
161.1 Nunn   p 128–129
162.1 Goodman & Gilman   p 416–417

161a) T Reflex pulmonary vasoconstriction is a phenomenon which occurs in the pulmonary circulation whereby hypoxia at a local level will cause vasoconstriction and thus reduce 'wasted' blood supply. The factors affecting this mechanism are varied. Both chemical and physical apply. Oxygen by definition prevents this response (161.1).

b) T Alpha adrenergic agonists cause pulmonary vasoconstriction. Tolazoline is an alpha blocking agent so it may reduce the effect of reflex vasoconstriction but will not necessarily abolish it. Be cautious here. It may be best to leave this question as a 'don't know' (161.1). The authors' opinion is a 'true' response.

c) F Adrenaline, which has a predominantly alpha effect, will accentuate reflex pulmonary vasoconstriction (161.1). This is detailed above.

d) F Almitrine has been noted to enhance reflex pulmonary vasoconstriction. This drug has been used mainly to increase the drive from peripheral chemoreceptors (161.1).

e) F The effect of hypercapnia is to reinforce hypoxic pulmonary vasoconstriction (161.1).

162a) F Many substances are contraindicated in patients on monoamine oxidase inhibitor (MAOI) treatment but butter is not listed among them (162.1).

b) T MAOIs interfere with the metabolism of amines. Problems arise when the precursors of biogenic amines are administered concomitantly. 5-hydroxytryptamine is an example. The major problem which occurs is a large release of noradrenaline which can lead to a hypertensive crisis. With respect to cheese it is aged cheese which causes most trouble due to the high content of tyramine. The tyramine escapes oxidative deamination in the liver and causes release of noradrenaline which is present in abnormally high amounts in nerve endings (162.1).

c) F Exogenously administered catecholamines are destroyed by COMT (catechyl-o-methyl-transferase) and not monoamine oxidase (162.1).

d) T Amphetamines act peripherally, mainly by releasing stored catecholamine at nerve endings. Profound potentiation of their pressor effects occurs (162.1).

e) T The adverse effect is due to the high tyramine content of chianti (an Italian red wine) (162.1).

163 No apologies are made for including a second question on MAOI drugs. The perspective is a little different to the preceding one.

Concurrent MAOI therapy will interfere with the action of the following drugs:
a) perphenazine
b) ephedrine
c) levodopa
d) dopamine
e) pethidine

164 For any practising anaesthetist it is advisable to memorize those agents which will provoke enzyme induction in the porphyrias. This is a very common topic in the clinical section of the FCAnaes Part 3 examination.

The following drugs are contraindicated in acute intermittent porphyria:
a) thiopentone
b) propofol
c) sulphonamides
d) diazepam
e) morphine

References

163.1	BNF	appendix 1
163.2	Dundee, Clarke & McCaughey	p 563–564
164.1	Aitkenhead & Smith	p 675
164.2	BNF	section 9.8.2
164.3	Nimmo & Smith	p 789

163a) F There is no interaction between phenothiazines (to which group perphenazine belongs) and MAOI drugs. Note that perphenazine does not feature in the detailed list of interactions with MAOIs in the BNF (163.1).

b) T Ephedrine causes hypertensive crisis in a manner similar to amphetamine. All indirectly acting sympathomimetics (to which class ephedrine belongs) may have an accentuated action. The effects of MAOI administration are complex. CNS monoamines do increase but synthesis falls. The false transmitter octopamine is formed and there may be initial stimulation of dopaminergic and presynaptic alpha receptors. Longer treatment causes a reduction in number and sensitivity of adrenergic and serotoninergic receptors with little effect on the dopamine receptor population. In summary there is a general reduction in sympathetic tone (163.2).

c) T Levodopa and other dopaminergic agents cause hypertensive crises (163.1).

d) T Monoamine oxidase may be categorized into two types, A and B. MAO-A is responsible for the metabolism of the monoamines. The response to dopamine is greatly exaggerated and hypertensive crises may occur (163.1).

e) T Pethidine is a classic example of a potential problem when mixed with MAOI drugs. The reduced ability to metabolize pethidine results in hypotension and coma. A hyperpyrexic reaction may be seen, thought to result from the release of 5-HT, an effect which may apply to other opioid analgesics (163.2). Analgesics which have been used uneventfully in this situation include pentazocine, morphine, and fentanyl.

164a) T This is fundamental. The porphyrias are a group of inherited conditions involving a disturbance of porphyrin metabolism in which there is a characteristic increase in the activity of gamma amino laevulinic acid synthetase which causes excessive output of porphyrins. Any agent which causes induction of this enzyme is contraindicated and the barbiturates are a good example (164.1).

b) F Although it is still early days propofol is not contraindicated in the acute porphyrias (164.1). Views may change with experience.

c) T Sulphonamides as a group are contraindicated (this includes trimethoprim and sulphasalazine) (164.2).

d) F Diazepam is quoted as an agent which is safe for use in porphyria (164.3).

e) F Morphine will not precipitate porphyria and is considered safe in this situation (164.3).

165 The concept of prodrugs and their actions is necessary to answer this. A definition of a prodrug would be advantageous (165.1).

The following are examples of prodrugs:
a) suxamethonium
b) diamorphine
c) gallamine
d) L-dopa
e) enalapril

166 Hepatic enzyme induction is a clinical problem. It is necessary to know the wide range of drugs which may cause enzyme induction and not just the group of commonly used anaesthetic agents.

Enzyme induction is a feature of:
a) ethyl alcohol
b) nitrazepam
c) enflurane
d) cimetidine
e) rifampicin

References
165.1 Vickers, Morgan & Spencer   p 26
165.2 Vickers, Morgan & Spencer   p 270
165.3 Goodman & Gilman   p 498
165.4 Dundee, Clarke & McCaughey   p 274
165.5 Vickers, Morgan & Spencer   p 232–233
165.6 Data Sheet Compendium   p 921

166.1 Calvey & Williams   p 24
166.2 Calvey & Williams   p 25
166.3 Goodman & Gilman   p 354
166.4 Rang & Dale   p 828–829

165a) F Prodrugs are pharmacologically inactive precursors which are metabolized into active components. A frequently quoted example is the conversion of chloral to trichloroethanol (which does not appear in this question!) (165.1). It can be difficult to decide whether a drug is a prodrug if parent and metabolite both have pharmacological activity. In considering your responses be guided as to whether an agent is a prodrug by the <u>necessity</u> of its conversion to an active agent. Suxamethonium itself is active and is metabolized to largely inactive metabolites (165.2). The monocholine has a minor neuromuscular blocking effect of its own. This is only about 5% of the parental activity.

b) T Diamorphine is hydrolysed into 6-monoacetyl morphine (6-MAM) then to morphine in vivo (165.3). Morphine and 6-MAM are responsible for the pharmacological effects of diamorphine.

c) F Gallamine is active itself. A lesser used competitive muscle relaxant, gallamine is characterized by the nature of its excretion which is almost entirely renal (165.4).

d) T L-dopa (levodopa) is deliberately given to enable penetration of the blood brain barrier after which it is converted to its active element dopamine (165.5).

e) T Following oral administration enalapril is rapidly absorbed and hydrolysed to enalaprilat, a highly specific, long acting non-sulphydryl angiotensin converting enzyme (165.6).

166a) T Enzyme induction is a feature of alcohol intake especially on a chronic basis (166.1). Acute intoxication with alcohol will, however, inhibit hepatic microsomal enzymes in man (166.2). Nevertheless induction is a feature of alcohol intake.

b) F Benzodiazepines do not cause significant induction of hepatic microsomal enzyme synthesis (166.3).

c) T All the anaesthetic vapours cause enzyme induction which contributes to the degree of their metabolism (166.1). This characteristic varies between agents and is most marked with respect to halothane.

d) F Cimetidine is a potent <u>inhibitor</u> of enzymes. Watch out! (166.2).

e) T Rifampicin is a well known enzyme inducer (166.4). Still used in the treatment of tuberculosis it has declined in popularity.

167 It is crucial to know which drugs cross the placenta and blood–brain barrier and the principles that underly the permeability of these barriers. The placenta is a modified lipid membrane across which drug passage is mainly governed by lipid solubility.

The following cross the placental membrane:
a) vecuronium
b) enflurane
c) suxamethonium
d) methohexitone
e) alfentanil

168 Local anaesthesia is a frequent topic. Following the stem very simple completions may be combined with taxing completions that need an extremely detailed knowledge of these agents. Questions on local anaesthetic agents often occur in vivas. A favourite is toxic doses of the various drugs with and without the addition of adrenaline. Learn those doses.

Bupivacaine:
a) inhibits excitatory cells within the brain
b) reduces action potentials
c) reduces calcium flux across membranes
d) is strongly protein bound
e) is more effective in acidic media

References

167.1 Atkinson, Rushman & Lee   p 267
167.2 Vickers, Morgan & Spencer   p 18
167.3 Data Sheet Compendium   p 788
167.4 Data Sheet Compendium   p 658

168.1 Vickers, Morgan & Spencer   p 203–204
168.2 Calvey & Williams   p 241–242

167a) F Vecuronium does not cross the placenta. Vecuronium is commonly used in Caesarean sections where such transfer would be undesirable to say the least (167.1).

b) T Inhalational anaesthetics and thiopentone rapidly attain equilibrium with fetal blood after administration to the mother (167.2).

c) F Highly ionized drugs of low lipid solubility such as suxamethonium and the non-depolarizing muscle relaxants, penetrate the placenta but this is an extremely slow process (167.2).

d) T Passage of methohexitone across both the placenta and blood–brain barrier is rapid because of its high lipid solubility and lack of protein binding (167.3).

e) T Alfentanil should not be given to the mother before the clamping of the cord during Caesarean section due to the possibility of respiratory depression in the newborn infant (167.4). Morphine, pethidine, and most other opioid analgesics readily pass to the fetus (167.2).

168a) T All local anaesthetic agents can penetrate the blood–brain barrier and produce a stabilizing effect on central neurones. It is therefore theoretically possible to control status epilepticus (if adequate doses are used). However, under normal conditions, inhibitory neurones are more sensitive to the actions of local anaesthetic agents than the excitatory neurones and thus excitatory events are more common (168.1). This is the root cause of the convulsions which are seen in local anaesthetic toxicity.

b) T Local anaesthetic agents act by preventing the depolarization of the axon. They do this by preventing the migration of ions across the nerve membrane. It is believed that local anaesthetic drugs compete with calcium ions at a receptor site which controls membrane permeability (168.1).

c) F Calcium ions are implicated in the mechanism of action of the local anaesthetic agents but not in respect of their flux across membranes (168.1).

d) T All the amide local anaesthetics are protein bound by up to 50%. In asscending order: lignocaine, mepivacaine and, most, bupivacaine (168.2).

e) F Once injected it is the amount of the drug in the form of the free base at the surrounding pH that is active. The amount of free base is determined by the pKa of the drug. If the pH is lowered (for example by inflammation) there is a great decrease in the amount of active free base present (168.1). The reverse situation also holds true. Alkalization of solutions of local anaesthetics to speed onset is well documented.

169 Prilocaine has gained popularity in intravenous regional anaesthesia due to its low toxicity compared to bupivacaine. The completions below could apply to ropivacaine (169.1) which would be more difficult to answer.

The following statements are true of prilocaine:
a) it is more potent than lignocaine
b) it may cause methaemoglobinaemia in large doses
c) it belongs to the ester group of local agents
d) it is the agent of choice in intravenous regional anaesthesia
e) it has pKa 7.9

170 The more newly introduced anaesthetic agents are an obvious area of interest to examiners. Regrettably there is usually a time lag between the introduction into practice and incorporation into textbooks. Look to the major journals for reviews on the agent. Product information supplied by manufacturers can be useful and other up-to-date sources can be found in both the 'Anaesthesia Review' series and 'Recent Advances'.

2, 6-Diisopropylphenol:
a) has a pH of 7
b) is more potent than thiopentone
c) undergoes rapid renal metabolism
d) is excreted unchanged by the kidney
e) releases histamine

References		
169.1 Anaesthesia (1991) 46	p 339–341
169.2 Erikson	p 12
169.3 BNF	section 15.2
169.4 Goodman & Gilman	p 390
169.5 Miller	p 1055
169.6 Dundee, Clarke & McCaughey	p 287
170.1 Dundee, Clarke & McCaughey	p 159
170.2 Diprivan®	p 10
170.3 Diprivan®	p 27
170.4 Diprivan®	p 9

169a) F The anaesthetic potency of prilocaine when applied to isolated nerves is lower than that of lignocaine (169.1).

b) T In high doses prilocaine is well known to cause methaemoglobinaemia. The treatment of methaemoglobinaemia is methylene blue 1%, 75–100 mg (169.2).

c) F Prilocaine is an amide not an ester (196.3).

d) T Due to its low level of toxicity when compared to its main rivals bupivacaine and lignocaine, prilocaine is the agent of choice in intravenous regional anaesthesia (169.4).

e) T Prilocaine has a pKa of 7.9 (169.5).

170a) T The pH of 2,6-diisopropylphenol (propofol) is relatively neutral and lies between 6 and 8.5. Note that the pKa of the drug in water is 11 (170.1).

b) T Propofol is about 1.8 times more potent than thiopentone (170.2).

c) F Propofol is highly lipophilic and rapidly metabolized in the liver, primarily to its inactive glucuronide conjugate and to the corresponding quinol together with its glucuronide conjugate. Inactive metabolites are excreted in the urine (170.3).

d) F Only inactive metabolites are excreted by the kidney (170.3). Occasional discolouration of urine has been reported.

e) F Propofol has not been shown to release histamine in animal models. Firm data on humans are sketchy at the time of writing (170.4). Whilst the emulsion formulation seems not to cause histamine release this was a feature of the agent in Cremophor® formulation. The role of drug and vehicle cannot be entirely separated in this context.

171 Following a recent change in the format of the London Part 2 FRCAnaes MCQ examination when certain groupings of questions appeared on the same topic, the authors felt it appropriate to emulate the style. Thus occasionally in this book juxtaposed questions on the same topic occur.

Propofol:
a) is a pale straw coloured liquid at room temperature
b) has a pKa of 11 in water
c) is formulated in soyabean oil
d) should be avoided in patients with disorders of fat metabolism
e) has a molecular weight of 178 Daltons

172 The physiology of pain transmission is confusing and detailed. The recent explosion of publications on opioid receptors keeps the topic very much in the public eye. Try to keep up with the journals.

With respect to opioid receptors:
a) mu receptors mediate spinal analgesia
b) kappa receptors are mainly found in the spinal cord
c) dynorphin is a kappa agonist
d) nalbuphine is an antagonist at mu receptors
e) sigma receptors are responsible for dysphoria

References
171.1 Diprivan®   p 7
171.2 Dundee, Clarke & McCaughey   p 159

172.1 BJA (1991) 66   p 370–380
172.2 Goodman & Gilman   p 488

171a) T Be careful here! Propofol is the approved name of 2,6-diisopropylphenol which is a straw coloured liquid at room temperature (171.1). The preparation of propofol for clinical use is an emulsion which has a white colour due to its constituents which are listed below.

b) T The pKa of propofol in water is 11 (171.2).

c) T The current preparation of propofol is a 1% aqueous emulsion which contains 10% w/v soyabean oil, 1.2% w/v egg phosphatide, and 2.25% w/v glycerol (171.2).

d) T Because of the formulation with a lipid emulsion it is advisable, although perhaps not essential, to avoid propofol in this situation (171.2).

e) T Either you know this or you don't! (171.1). The molecular weight of 2,6-diisopropylphenol is 178 Daltons.

172a) F Although mu receptors are most certainly intimately connected with analgesia their central location within the CNS implies an involvement with supraspinal analgesia. Mu receptors are widely distributed in areas of the brain associated with pain and sensorimotor integration. In contrast kappa receptors are mainly localized to the spinal cord and are linked with spinal analgesia per se (172.1). There is no known <u>selective</u> endogenous ligand for mu receptors.

b) T Kappa receptors are predominantly found in the spinal cord. Note the comments above (172.1).

c) T Dynorphin is the endogenous ligand at kappa receptors (172.1).

d) T Nalbuphine shows the unusual feature of receptor dualism. This is represented by the fact that it has agonal activity at kappa sites but antagonal activity at mu sites (172.2).

e) T The sigma receptor is implicated in the psychotomimetic effects of opioids (172.1). Strictly speaking, as sigma agonists are not reversed by naloxone, sigma is not an opioid receptor. The sigma receptor may be the phenylcyclohexylpiperidine receptor which is associated with ketamine and phencyclidine.

173 To answer questions on pharmacokinetics a sound understanding of the subject and logical thinking are required. The subject is inescapable so it is therefore important to have a clear mind that will resist any doubts that the questions may generate.

First order kinetics:
a) are the most common kinetics encountered in drug metabolism
b) multiple doses result in a steady state when first order kinetics apply
c) can only occur in a single compartment model
d) show the saturation phenomenon
e) are represented by alcohol

174 The general pharmacology sections of most of the major texts carry revision material on agonist/antagonist definitions. Do not skip these sections when revising.

Non-competitive antagonists:
a) move log dose–response curve to the right in a non-parallel manner
b) reduce the gradient of the log dose–response curve
c) have a response unrelated to their plasma concentration
d) prevent a maximum agonal response
e) have a long duration of action

References	
173.1 Rang & Dale	p 106
173.2 Rang & Dale	p 100–102
173.3 Rang & Dale	p 102–106
174.1 Calvey & Williams	p 92–93

173a) T First order kinetics are the most commonly encountered; however, some drugs may obey zero order kinetics (173.1).

b) T When first order kinetics apply, multiple doses or infusion of a drug result in a rising concentration until a steady state is reached such that mean rate of administration is equal to mean rate of elimination (173.2).

c) F First order kinetics relate both to single and multiple compartment models (173.3).

d) T The saturation phenomenon occurs with drugs that obey first order kinetics (173.1). Saturation kinetics describe a change from first to zero order elimination.

e) F Ethanol obeys zero order kinetics, that is to say its rate of excretion is independent of plasma concentration and proceeds at a constant rate (173.1). Make sure that you remember this definition.

174a) T Non-competitive agonists compose a group whose effects cannot be entirely explained by a simple process of competition with an agonist. It is usual for a stable chemical bond to be formed between drug and receptor. The log dose–response curve is usually shifted to the right in a non-parallel manner (that is to say there is a change in the gradient of the curve) and the subsequent attainment of a maximum agonal response is prevented (174.1).

b) T The gradient of the log dose–response curve is reduced by non-competitive antagonists (174.1).

c) T Non-competitive antagonists usually have an effect unrelated to plasma concentration. It is the concentration at the biophase that is the most important feature (174.1).

d) T Maximum agonal response will be prevented; indeed this is a sensible definition of an antagonist in its own right (174.1).

e) T This is a corollary of the strong chemical bond described above. That is why a long duration of action is common with this group of drugs (174.1).

175 Several groups of drugs may interfere with the metabolism of both vitamin B_{12} and folic acid. This may occur by a variety of mechanisms.

The following drugs interfere with folate metabolism:
a) sulphonamides
b) trimethoprim
c) sodium nitroprusside
d) penicillin
e) nitrous oxide

176 Non-steroidal anti-inflammatory agents are widely prescribed. They comprise a huge group and unfortunately the wide scope may lead to some confusion. The various marketed agents have a propensity for appearing and disappearing with regularity which makes it difficult to keep up to date.

Non-steroidal anti-inflammatory drugs:
a) should not be used in hypertensive patients
b) reduce platelet stickiness
c) increase the effect of warfarin
d) are available in parenteral form
e) affect prostaglandin synthesis

References

175.1 Rang & Dale   p 807
175.2 Rang & Dale   p 809–810
175.3 Dundee, Clarke & McCaughey   p 386–390
175.4 Rang & Dale   p 813
175.5 Recent Advances 16   p 33

176.1 BNF   section 10.1.1
176.2 Atkinson, Rushman & Lee   p 121
176.3 Rang & Dale   p 117
176.4 BJA (1990) 65   p 445–447
176.5 Rang & Dale   p 284–285

175a) T Sulphonamides have a bacteriostatic action which results from competition with para-amino benzoic acid for the enzyme dihydropteroate synthetase. The net result of this is a disturbance of folate synthesis. Bacteria must synthesize folate but in humans it is dietarily sourced (175.1).

b) T Trimethoprim interferes with dihydrofolate reductase and is thus a folate antagonist (175.2).

c) F The effect of nitroprusside is not connected with folate. Rather, nitroprusside is broken down by haemoglobin non-enzymatically (175.3).

d) F Penicillin acts by obstructing the synthesis of the bacterial cell wall peptidoglycan (175.4). It has no effect on folate metabolism.

e) T Nitrous oxide causes inactivation of B_{12} when administered for long periods. The resultant inhibition of methionine synthetase blocks the conversion of methyl tetrahydro folate to tetrahydro folate (175.5).

176a) F Although there may be a theoretical risk to hypertensive patients from the retention of sodium which is a feature of this group of drugs, hypertension is not listed as a contraindication to NSAID therapy (176.1).

b) T A reduction in platelet stickiness is an effect of NSAIDs (176.2). This is an action which may have clinical significance.

c) T This effect is due to the displacement of warfarin from protein binding sites (176.3) which increases the unbound fraction.

d) T The newer agents, for example ketorolac, are recommended for parenteral use (176.4). Ketorolac is available in oral and parenteral preparations.

e) T The effect of NSAIDs on prostaglandin synthesis is the inhibition of cyclo-oxygenase, the enzyme that is responsible for the conversion of arachidonic acid to prostaglandin endoperoxidases (176.5). That enzyme inhibition is the basis for their clinical effects.

177 Questions on antibiotics may be difficult to answer as these drugs are seldom prescribed by anaesthetists, although they are often given on induction of anaesthesia by surgical request. Administration of antibiotics on induction has been criticized due to the potential for obscuring the cause of anaphylaxis related to anaesthetic drugs.

Tetracycline:
a) is active against Gram positive and Gram negative organisms
b) causes necrotizing enterocolitis
c) does not cross the blood–brain barrier
d) can enter bone
e) should not be taken during pregnancy

178 When a drug is used as an antagonist it is important to differentiate between the effects that occur as a result of reversal of the agonist and those which can be directly attributed to the drug itself.

Naloxone:
a) produces dysphoria
b) can cause pulmonary oedema
c) reverses pentazocine
d) causes a rise in blood pressure
e) is an H_2 agonist

References
177.1 Rang & Dale   p 817–818
177.2 BNF   section 5.1.3
177.3 Oxford Textbook of Medicine   section 5. 274–277

178.1 Goodman & Gilman   p 515
178.2 Atkinson, Rushman & Lee   p 132
178.3 Data Sheet Compendium   p 433
178.4 BJA (1985) 57   p 547–550
178.5 Rang & Dale   p 258–261

177a) T The tetracyclines are active against a very wide spectrum of micro-organisms including Gram positive and Gram negative bacteria, *Mycoplasma rickettsia, Chlamydia, Brucella*, and some protozoa. Their mechanism of action is inhibition of protein synthesis after uptake into susceptible organisms by active transport. Tetracyclines are bacteriostatic (177.1).

b) F Beware, tetracyclines have been reported to cause pseudomembranous colitis (177.2), a disease due to colonization of the colon with *Clostridium difficile* (177.3). Necrotizing enterocolitis is caused by *Clostridium perfringens* (welchii) and is sometimes called gas gangrene of the gut (177.3). Do not confuse these two conditions.

c) F Tetracyclines have a wide distribution in the body. They enter most compartments and cross the blood–brain barrier and placenta. Tetracyclines also appear in breast milk (177.1).

d) T Tetracyclines chelate calcium and are deposited in growing bones and teeth, resulting in staining and sometimes dental hypoplasia and bone deformities. Therefore they should never be given to children, pregnant women, or nursing mothers (177.1).

e) T Fetal bone and dental damage can occur. This is described above (177.1).

178a) F In the absence of opioid drugs naloxone is almost devoid of agonistic effects. In man doses of up to 12 mg produce no discernible subjective effects and even 24 mg produce only slight drowsiness. Oral doses of more than 1 g have been given without any major subjective or physiological effects (178.1).

b) T Naloxone has caused acute pulmonary oedema in a previously fit adult (178.2). The underlying pathophysiology of this is not understood. Possibly it is the result of acute CNS activity due to sudden opioid reversal.

c) T Naloxone may be used for complete or partial reversal of opioid effects induced by natural and synthetic opioids and the agonist–antagonists such as nalbuphine pentazocine or dextropropoxyphene (178.3).

d) F In normal man there is no change in blood pressure. See above (178.1). However, beware, naloxone may raise blood pressure in septic shock (a pathological state) (178.2). There is a great deal of debate over the possible mechanisms associated with this effect (178.4).

e) F The histamine receptor system is different and there is no cross reactivity (178.5). This is another distractor.

179 MAC is a useful practical index which has its own definition. MAC values for the commonly used vapours are often asked as are those for agents of historical interest.

The MAC of an inhalational anaesthetic agent:
a) is the maximum allowable concentration that can be given safely
b) must be determined in unpremedicated subjects
c) is determined by measuring the inspired concentration of an agent
d) indicates when 50% of a population will not move when a surgical incision is made
e) is used to indicate equipotent concentrations of inhalational agents

180 The provision of anaesthesia for pregnant and recently delivered patients requires detailed knowledge of the effects of anaesthetic agents on uterine contractility. Note the phrase 'clinical concentrations' in the stem.

The following drugs in clinical concentrations will cause uterine relaxation:
a) cyclopropane
b) thiopentone
c) trichloroethylene
d) ether
e) halothane

References
179.1 Miller   p 53
179.2 Aitkenhead & Smith   p 154
179.3 Nimmo & Smith   p 36

180.1 Dundee, Clarke & McCaughey   p 132
180.2 Vickers, Morgan & Spencer   p 72
180.3 Vickers, Morgan & Spencer   p 155–157
180.4 Vickers, Morgan & Spencer   p 158
180.5 Dundee, Clarke & McCaughey   p 118–119

179a) F In 1963 Mekel and Eger described the minimal alveolar concentration of an agent which at 1 atmosphere abolished movement of 50% of a population in response to a noxious stimulus. MAC 1.0 was defined as the minimal alveolar concentration of anaesthetic required to keep a dog from responding by gross purposeful movement to a painful stimulus. This concept has led to its use as a comparison of anaesthetic potency between agents. All the vapours are commonly delivered at 1–2 MAC in clinical situations (179.1).

b) T MAC is determined in unpremedicated subjects and is reduced by the presence of premedication agents (179.2).

c) F Inspired concentration is not relevant. It is the end tidal concentration which is held constant over a 15 min period after which response to surgical skin incision is recorded (179.3).

d) T In humans the noxious stimulus is a surgical skin incision (179.1).

e) T MAC is the best comparative estimate of volatile anaesthetic potency (179.1).

180a) T Cyclopropane depresses uterine contractility in direct relationship with inspired concentration (180.1). The effect is slight but present at normal clinical concentrations of the agent.

b) F Thiopentone has little effect on uterine tone in low doses. At higher doses it may cause uterine relaxation (180.2).

c) F There is little effect of trichloroethylene on the uterus when used in analgesic concentrations. Higher inspired concentrations will cause relaxation of uterine muscle (180.3).

d) T This is a well known feature of ether in clinical concentrations and it is marked at deep levels of ether anaesthesia (180.4).

e) T Halothane causes uterine relaxation even at low concentrations (180.5). In higher concentrations the effect is marked.

181 Dopamine has different pharmacological actions which depend on the rate of infusion. The units used in the question may differ from those that you are used to. There is no room for discussion in MCQ answers.

Dopamine infusion at 10 μg/kg min^{-1}:
a) increases heart rate
b) reduces peripheral vascular resistance
c) increases renal blood flow
d) increases cardiac output
e) increases urine output

182 The welcome appearance of a question which appears to have a clinical bias is often offset by the realization that it doesn't. Clonidine is little used for the treatment of hypertension these days. Do not guess.

A patient on clonidine presenting for anaesthesia:
a) should not have received the most recent dose
b) may have postural hypotension
c) should not receive a noradrenaline infusion
d) should not receive a dopamine infusion
e) should not receive beta blockers

References

181.1 Aitkenhead & Smith   p 231

182.1 Dundee, Clarke & McCaughey   p 422
182.2 BNF   appendix 1

181a) F Tachycardia is a common effect of infusions which exceed 15 µg/kg min⁻¹. In lower doses the chronotropic effect of dopamine is minimal (181.1).

b) F A major effect of dopamine is the alpha adrenoceptor mediated effect of vasoconstriction which increases peripheral vascular resistance (181.1).

c) T The dose range over which dopamine has an effective action on the reduction of resistance in the renal vascular bed is 5–10 µg/kg min⁻¹. At higher doses widespread vasoconstriction will be the rule (181.1).

d) T Cardiac output at this dose level is increased by a direct inotropic action on the myocardium mediated by beta receptors (181.1).

e) T The urine output will be increased by a combination of increased cardiac output and increased renal blood flow as described above (181.1).

182a) F It is important not to withdraw clonidine abruptly prior to anaesthesia because rebound hypertension occurs (182.1). This completion aims at this very topic. Clonidine increases the storage of catecholamines within nerve terminals by an action of pre-synaptic alpha receptors. If clonidine is abruptly withdrawn these catecholamines are released. Ideally other hypotensive agents should be substituted for clonidine before anaesthesia.

b) F Clonidine is unusual with respect to other hypotensive agents in that normal cardiovascular homeostasis is maintained. Postural hypotension would only occur if it were a feature of the pathological process itself (182.1).

c) T Patients are normally extremely sensitive to the effects of both exogenous and endogenous catecholamines. This response may be open to some interpretation since reduced doses may be used safely (182.1).

d) T The situation with regard to dopamine is entirely analogous to that with regard to noradrenaline. See above (182.1).

e) T Beta blockers will potentiate the effects of clonidine withdrawal (182.2).

183 Diuretics are widely used drugs. Frequently patients will present for surgery receiving regular diuretic therapy, a probability which will increase with age. Knowledge of their detailed pharmacology will not be wasted. The two questions which follow involve thiazides which are waning in popularity with clinicians.

Long term administration of thiazide diuretics may be accompanied by:
a) hyperuricaemia
b) hypochloraemia
c) weight loss
d) hyponatraemia
e) metabolic alkalosis

184 Although used less today than previously, the thiazides provided the mainstay of diuretic therapy for many years before the arrival of the potent loop diuretics.

The thiazide diuretics:
a) greatly increase glomerular filtration rate
b) potentiate cardiac glycosides
c) may lessen polyuria in diabetes mellitus
d) may cause acute pancreatitis
e) may cause acute pulmonary oedema

References

183.1	BNF	section 2.2.1
183.2	Rang & Dale	p 434–435
184.1	Goodman & Gilman	p 719
184.2	BNF	section 2.1.1
184.3	Goodman & Gilman	p 721
184.4	Rang & Dale	p 435

183a) T Hyperuricaemia is a common occurrence during thiazide treatment and may even lead to clinical gout (183.1).
   b) T Hypochloraemia and hypokalaemia are well documented side effects of the thiazides and may be complicated by an associated alkalosis (183.1).
   c) T Weight loss is an obvious corollary of diuretic therapy and reduction of oedema although it may be an early and temporary event (183.1).
   d) T Thiazide diuretics may lead to hyponatraemia which can cause neurological signs (183.1). The process by which natriuresis occurs has not been explained.
   e) T The alkalosis which is seen in thiazide therapy is usually hypochloraemic alkalosis (183.2).

184a) F Far from greatly increasing glomerular filtration rate (GFR) the thiazide diuretics may actually cause a reduction in GFR. This effect is thought to be mediated by a direct action on renal vasculature (184.1).
   b) T That hypokalaemia potentiates the effects of cardiac glycosides is well known (184.2). All thiazides can produce hypokalaemia (184.1).
   c) F The paradoxical effects of the thiazides on urine volume apply to diabetes insipidus not diabetes mellitus (184.3). This is a classic distractor. Do not fall into such traps.
   d) T The unwanted effects of thiazides occur rarely but they are numerous and include pulmonary oedema and pancreatitis (184.1).
   e) T Pulmonary oedema can occur although this is not common. Other unwanted effects include dermatitis and blood dyscrasias (184.4).

185 Chelation is a physical effect which may be useful in the drug treatment of pathological conditions. One of the best known chelating agents is ethylenediaminetetraacetic acid (EDTA) which unfortunately does not appear in this question.

The following drugs may be used as chelators:
a) oxytetracycline
b) cobalt edetate
c) clioquinol
d) penicillin
e) desferrioxamine

186 From an area of drug action this question moves along to the vexed subject of pharmacokinetics. Consider each completion separately and try not to 'freeze' when daunted by an unpopular topic.

The following statements are true:
a) the Hill plot relates the log drug dose to log drug effect
b) the plasma half life of a drug is related to clearance and volume of distribution
c) total body clearance is the sum of clearances in organs which eliminate a drug
d) the kinetics of most intravenous drugs are consistent with two compartment kinetics
e) saturation kinetics are described by the Michaelis–Menten equation.

References

185.1 Calvey & Williams	p 73–74
186.1 Calvey & Williams	p 71
186.2 Calvey & Williams	p 38
186.3 Calvey & Williams	p 39–42
186.4 Calvey & Williams	p 54
186.5 Calvey & Williams	p 61–63

185a) T Chelating agents combine chemically with certain metallic ions and this feature can be used to remove elements from the body or may be an unwanted side effect. The tetracyclines are potent chelating agents which readily combine with iron, calcium, magnesium and aluminium ions. When such a combination is given orally the absorption of both ions and antibiotics may be impeded. The chelation of calcium and magnesium by tetracyclines may be part of the reason for their bacteriostatic effect (185.1).

b) T Cobalt edetate is used for the chelation of cyanide ions in cyanide poisoning and it can also be used to chelate cyanide ions from excess sodium nitroprusside therapy. Cobalt edetate is toxic and cyanide poisoning must be definite before the start of treatment (185.1).

c) T Clioquinol is sometimes used in the treatment of amoebic dysentery and may function by chelation of copper, iron and other heavy metals (185.1).

d) F Penicillin is not a chelating agent. It may be confused with penicillamine (185.1).

e) T Desferrioxamine is a specific chelating agent used in the treatment of iron toxicity and haemachromatosis. Desferrioxamine has a high affinity for iron bound to ferritin and haemosiderin (185.1).

186a) T The Hill plot relates the log of drug dose or concentration (x axis) to the value log $E/(E_{max}-E)$ (y axis). E is the response obtained at different dose levels and E_{max} the maximum effect observed. It is the linear relationship displayed by a Hill plot that simplifies statistical analysis (186.1).

b) T Plasma half life depends on both volume of distribution and clearance in the manner $T_{1/2}$ is proportional to V_D/Cl where V_D is volume of distribution and Cl is clearance (186.2).

c) T This is the classic definition of total body clearance (186.3). The answer is entirely logical and should not have proved difficult.

d) T The two compartment model which results commonly in the biexponential decline in initial plasma concentration fits the majority of intravenously administered drugs (186.4).

e) T Saturation kinetics describe a change from first order to a zero order process. This is consistent with Michaelis–Menten kinetics and the metabolic reactions are described by the Michaelis–Menten equation (186.5).

187 Desensitization, tachyphylaxis, and tolerance can all describe the same event under different circumstances.

The repeated use of a drug:
a) in the case of suxamethonium results in tachyphylaxis
b) may result in desensitization in the presence of autoimmune disorders
c) may result in endocytosis of receptors
d) can produce a decrease in the observed response due to a change in metabolism
e) can only produce desensitization in vivo

188 The half life (elimination half life) of a drug is a characteristic of a drug that helps the user to handle the drug effectively. This has direct relevance with respect to the half lives of the more important anaesthetic drugs.

The following statements are true:
a) half life is a hybrid value
b) half life can only be measured from initial concentration
c) drug doses are best given at intervals of twice their half life
d) drugs given by intravenous infusions reach steady state concentrations after 4–5 half lives
e) diazepam has a half life of 3000 min

References

187.1 Calvey & Williams   p 96–97
187.2 Aitkenhead & Smith   p 218

188.1 Calvey & Williams   p 42
188.2 Vickers, Morgan & Spencer   p 30
188.3 Dundee, Clarke & McCaughey   p 45

187a) T Tachyphylaxis can be described as a rapid progressive decrease in response to a drug and is sometimes described as acute desensitization or rapid tolerance. It can be observed after administration of tyramine, ephedrine or amphetamine (187.1). Tachyphylaxis can also occur when suxamethonium is given in repeated doses or as an infusion (187.2). Desensitization is a decrease in cellular sensitivity or responsiveness due to the continuous or repeated exposure to agonists. Tolerance is a chronic phenomenon in which increasing drug dose is required to produce the desired therapeutic effect (187.1). These are very important distinctions.

b) T Repeated use of a drug can lead to desensitization. Chronic desensitization due to receptor losses may occur with autoimmune processes, such as myasthenia gravis (187.1).

c) T Chronic desensitization is associated with loss of receptors due to reasons such as irreversible conformational changes, receptor degradation, or endocytosis (internalization) of receptors (187.1).

d) T In tolerance the reduction in response may occur because of receptor loss, chronic desensitization or increased metabolism (for example due to the induction of hepatic enzymes producing tolerance to barbiturates) (187.1).

e) F Desensitization is a phenomenon which is often observed in vitro. It is usually observed in isolated tissues or cell preparations (187.1).

188a) T Half life depends on other primary pharmacokinetic values and is therefore a hybrid value (188.1).

b) F Half life is the time required to eliminate 50% of the amount of drug that was present when the measurement was initiated (188.2).

c) F Drugs are usually best given at intervals approximately equal to their half lives. This applies to oral, intramuscular or intravenous routes. Drugs will then cumulate for 4–5 doses until steady state concentrations are reached (188.1).

d) T To within 5%, steady state concentrations are reached after 4–5 half lives of an infusion (188.1).

e) F The figure of 3000 min sets out to confuse. This is 50 h. The half life of diazepam is age dependent and varies between 75 h in the perinate and 18 h in the child. For adults, which is the assumed group considered in this question, the range is 20–42 h (188.3).

30–70hr?

189 Statistics are not generally the most popular topic for revision. Whilst the topic generates instinctive dislike there is nonetheless an important application of statistical principles to data handling. This is relevant to the design and execution of clinical trials.

With respect to statistics:
a) the null hypothesis states that there is no real difference between two sets of data
b) rejection of the null hypothesis leads to the acceptance of the alternate hypothesis
c) if the null hypothesis is wrongly rejected alpha error is present
d) beta error states that the null hypothesis has been wrongly accepted
e) the power of a study may be increased by raising the number of observations

190 The knowledge of statistics required to answer the question below is very elementary. Be certain that you possess it.

The following statements are true:
a) the mean is the arithmetic sum of the observations divided by their number
b) the median is the observation with half the observations above it and half below it
c) the mode is the most commonly occurring observation
d) the interquartile range embraces 25–75% of values
e) a large spread of data about the mean will result in a large variance

References

189.1 Scurr, Feldman & Soni   p 660–661

190.1 Scurr, Feldman & Soni   p 660–661

189a) T The null hypothesis is deliberately constructed to test the validity of a recorded difference between two sets of data. It says 'there is no real difference and any difference found must be due to chance' (189.1).

b) T If the null hypothesis is rejected then the assumption will be that there is a real difference. Thus the alternate hypothesis is adopted and this states that there is a real difference which is not due to chance (189.1).

c) T If the null hypothesis is wrongly rejected then a real difference has been missed and attributed to random chance. This form of error is referred to as alpha type (189.1). *Type 1*

d) T This is the opposite situation to that above (189.1). Beta error occurs when a difference is found that is actually due to chance. *Type II*

e) T The power of any test is a measure of the ability to recognize a difference when one is present. For a given level of alpha error raising the number of observations will increase the power (189.1).

190a) T This is a very elementary point. The definition of the mean in this completion is correct (190.1).

b) T This is the definition of the median. Note that when the number of observations is an even number the median will be the value between the two middle ranks (190.1).

c) T This is the definition of the mode (190.1).

d) T Quartiles are a useful way of describing a range and the inter-quartile range will embrace 25–75% of values (190.1).

e) T A wide variation of data about the mean results in both a high variance and a large standard deviation (190.1).

191 New drugs take some time to percolate into standard textbooks. Sources of information of an up-to-date nature are mostly journals and reviews. Flecainide has been publicized with respect to the cardiac arrhythmia suppression trial (CAST).

Flecainide:
a) is indicated in supraventricular arrhythmias
b) markedly increases QRS duration
c) may be given orally
d) is a negative inotrope
e) has a narrow therapeutic range

192 The classification of the antiarrhythmic agents is absolutely essential knowledge for the examination. A helpful cardiologist might be cajoled into a tutorial on the subject. A personal revision table is useful.

With regard to antiarrhythmic agents:
a) class I drugs block sodium channels
b) class III drugs prolong the refractory period of the myocardium
c) lignocaine belongs to class I
d) beta blockers belong to more than one group
e) class I drugs have a wide variety of clinical applications

References
191.1 Dundee, Clarke & McCaughey   p 376
191.2 Lancet (1989) 55   p 481–483
191.3 Bennett   p 113
191.4 Goodman & Gilman   p 861–864

192.1 Rang & Dale   p 330–335

191a) F Oral preparations are used for chronic prophylaxis of ventricular tachyarrhythmias, unifocal and multifocal ventricular extrasystoles, and A–V nodal reciprocating tachycardia (Wolff–Parkinson–White syndrome). Absorption of flecainide is prompt and complete after oral administration. Intravenous preparations are suitable for acute control of ventricular tachycardia and Wolff–Parkinson–White syndrome (191.1) (191.2).

b) T Flecainide is in class Ic of the Vaughan Williams classification, i.e. it is an agent which does not affect the duration of the action potential (191.1). The action potential is not identical to the QRS complex and QRS duration is increased (191.1).

c) T Oral doses of 100–300 mg twice daily are recommended (191.1).

d) T Systolic ejection fraction and myocardial contractility decrease, both contributing to a reduced cardiac output (191.3).

e) T The drug has a narrow therapeutic range, i.e. it can be difficult to achieve a therapeutic action without unwanted effects (191.3) (191.4).

192a) T Class I drugs block sodium channels in the same fashion as local anaesthetic agents. The characteristic effect of these drugs on the action potential is a reduction in the rate of depolarization during phase 0. Examples are quinidine, procainamide, lignocaine, and phenytoin (192.1).

b) T Class III drugs prolong the action potential and refractory period of the myocardium and therefore diminish the incidence of re-entrant rhythms. It is a poorly understood group that includes amiodarone and some beta receptor antagonists (192.1).

c) T Lignocaine is a class I agent used by infusion to suppress ventricular arrhythmias (192.1).

d) T Classically beta adrenergic receptor antagonists belong to class II. Beta blockers have other effects in addition to their actions on the sympathetic nervous system which means that they fulfil the criteria of some other classes (192.1).

e) T Class I drugs are featured above. They have a variety of differing clinical applications (192.1). This is illustrated by listing some members of this category, for example procainamide, disopyramide, phenytoin, and lignocaine. This enclave covers therapeutic doctrines from epilepsy to local anaesthesia.

193 Induction agents are the tools of our trade. Apparent ignorance of these agents in the MCQ will be a disadvantage and in a viva will give a very poor impression.

Etomidate:
a) is a carboxylated imidazole
b) is soluble in water
c) has a pH of 8.1
d) causes muscle movements which are associated with epileptiform changes on the EEG
e) is approximately 75% protein bound

194 Thiopentone remains the most widely used drug in anaesthesia although hotly pursued by propofol. There is no excuse for ignorance as the accumulated database on the drug is vast.

Thiopentone:
a) a 2.5% solution has a pH of 10.5
b) contains sodium carbonate
c) has a pKa of 7.6
d) reduces cerebral oxygen consumption
e) can enter red blood cells

References

193.1 Atkinson, Rushman & Lee   p 237–239

194.1 Atkinson, Rushman & Lee   p 229–230

193a) T Etomidate is a carboxylated imidazole (ethyl-1-(a-methyl-benzyl) medazole-5-carboxylate) (193.1).
b) T Etomidate is a white crystalline powder soluble in a wide range of solvents including water, ethanol, and propylene glycol. The commercial preparation consists of the drug dissolved in water with 35% propylene glycol (193.1).
c) T The pH of the commercial preparation is 8.1 (193.1).
d) F The EEG changes are similar to those seen with thiopentone. The muscle movements that are frequently seen during induction are not associated with epileptiform discharges, suggesting that the origin is in deep cerebral structures or the brain stem itself (193.1).
e) T In the blood, etomidate distributes equally between red blood cells and plasma and the protein binding is 76.5%. Only 2.5% can be found in the circulation 2 min after injection (193.1).

194a) T Thiopentone is soluble in water and alcohol and forms a 2.5% or 5% solution in water of pH 10.5 approximately (194.1).
b) T 6% anhydrous sodium carbonate is added to thiopentone to prevent formation of free acid by atmospheric carbon dioxide (194.1).
c) T The pKa value for thiopentone is 7.6. In acidosis the plasma levels of thiopentone fall by up to 40% with return to control values on return to normal pH (in experimental animals) (194.1). The importance of pKa for induction agents is related to their ability to cross membranes. Ideally, high lipid solubility will result in easy passage into neurolipid. A balance is necessary between lipid solubility and a degree of water solubility which enables easy formulation.
d) T Cerebral oxygen consumption is reduced. So are cerebral blood flow, CSF pressure, and intracranial pressure (194.1).
e) T Thiopentone enters red cells to reach a concentration of about 40% of that found in plasma (194.1).

195 Suxamethonium is the only depolarizing muscle relaxant used routinely in the UK. Other examples of this type of relaxant are available in other countries. Questions may relate to the pharmacokinetics and pharmacodynamics of those drugs as well as suxamethonium.

With regard to depolarizing muscle relaxants:
a) suxamethonium is stable for at least 14 days at room temperature
b) repeated doses can cause post-tetanic potentiation and tetanic fade
c) decamethonium can cause histamine release
d) pseudocholinesterase can be found in red cells
e) plasma cholinesterase deficiency can be caused by ketamine

196 The pharmacology of muscle relaxants and the physiology of the neuromuscular junction are linked topics of mutual application. Revising them together may be helpful.

Pancuronium:
a) may cause plasma cholinesterase deficiency
b) in solution has a pH of 7
c) is the relaxant of choice in atopic patients because of its steroidal activity
d) releases adrenaline from adrenergic nerve endings
e) is 80% protein bound

References	
195.1 Trissel	p 711–712
195.2 Miller	p 675
195.3 Atkinson, Rushman & Lee	p 275
195.4 Atkinson, Rushman & Lee	p 280
195.5 Atkinson, Rushman & Lee	p 276–277
196.1 Trissel	p 583
196.2 Current Anaesthesia and Critical Care (1989)1.1	p 43
196.3 Atkinson, Rushman & Lee	p 270

195a) T Although suxamethonium is stored between 2 and 8°C to retard potency loss, the drug is stable at room temperature for 14 days. Calculated loss of potency at room temperature is 1% per week. At 40°C ambient temperature it is 3.2% per week (195.1).

b) T Repeated doses of depolarizing relaxants such as suxamethonium and decamethonium alter the response at the neuromuscular junction. A phase II block occurs, the characteristics of which are tetanic fade, post-tetanic potentiation, train of four fade, and possible partial or complete reversal with edrophonium or neostigmine (195.2).

c) F Decamethonium does not release histamine (195.3). However, suxamethonium <u>does</u> release histamine leading to bronchospasm, hypotension, and acute circulatory collapse without previous exposure (195.4).

d) F Plasma cholinesterase is a lipoprotein synthesized in the liver. It is found in plasma but not in red cells. It is also found in the liver, brain, kidneys, and pancreas (195.5).

e) T There are a number of causes of abnormal metabolism of suxamethonium. These can be due to abnormal plasma cholinesterase (inherited), plasma cholinesterase deficiency, plasma cholinesterase antagonism, and plasma cholinesterase excess. Ketamine can cause plasma cholinesterase deficiency (195.5).

196a) T Pancuronium can produce an acquired plasma cholinesterase deficiency (195.5).

b) F Pancuronium is formulated in sodium acetate, benzyl alcohol, and sodium chloride for isotonicity. Acetic acid and/or sodium hydroxide is added to adjust the pH to 4 (196.1).

c) F Histamine release is not prominent and anaphylactoid reactions are very rare. Pancuronium is probably the relaxant of choice for the atopic individual (196.2). Pancuronium is a bis-quaternary aminosteroid which is devoid of hormonal activity (196.3). Thus although indicated in atopic patients this is <u>not</u> due to steroidal activity.

d) F Pancuronium produces a sympathomimetic effect via an indirect mechanism: it releases noradrenaline from adrenergic nerve endings (196.2).

e) T The plasma binding of pancuronium is about 80% and is unaffected by disease states (196.2).

197 Any particular drug within a class may be examined. Include as many as possible in your revision—even those which have fallen from grace. Gallamine is still stocked in many anaesthetic rooms.

The following statements are true of muscle relaxants:
a) gallamine will cross the placental barrier
b) gallamine has a pharmacologically active metabolite
c) diallyl nortoxiferine is miscible with methohexitone
d) alcuronium binds to serum albumin
e) the potency of gallamine decreases with an increase in pH.

198 Enquiring about clinical trials can exhibit a candidate's understanding of design and protocol. The subject can rapidly progress to statistical analysis of the results of any trial. Be warned.

In clinical trials:
a) a trial can be set up without a hypothesis
b) any trial should attempt to answer as many questions as possible
c) randomization between two groups is not essential
d) in a single blind study the subject does not know if an active agent or placebo is being administered
e) in a single blind study the investigator does not know if an active agent or placebo is being administered

References

197.1 Atkinson, Rushman & Lee   p 269–270
197.2 Vickers, Morgan & Spencer   p 263
197.3 Vickers, Morgan & Spencer   p 267

198.1 Scurr, Feldman & Soni   p 657–660

197a) T Gallamine passes the placental barrier and should not be used in obstetrics routinely although some workers do use the drug in Caesarean section (197.1).

b) T Between 15 and 40% of gallamine is degraded. The 3-hydroxy metabolite has about half the neuromuscular blocking activity of the parent drug. About 80% of the parent drug is renally excreted so the drug should not be used in patients with renal failure (197.1).

c) T Diallyl nortoxiferine is alcuronium! Alcuronium is miscible in the same syringe with methohexitone but not with thiopentone (197.1). The practice is not recommended.

d) T Alcuronium is mainly bound to serum albumin (197.2). A correlation may be seen between the dose requirement of a patient and the measured serum albumin.

e) F In man there is an increase in potency as pH increases. This is probably related to changes in binding to albumin (197.3).

198a) F At the centre of a trial is an idea, or hypothesis. The process used to examine an hypothesis is the experimental method of the scientific investigation (198.1).

b) F A clinical trial is designed to test the hypothesis and, depending on the result, the hypothesis is rejected, modified, or retained for further information. There is only one hypothesis per trial (198.1).

c) T Randomization is the process by which the subjects in a drug trial are allocated to receive either the study drug or the control and the allocation is governed by chance. There are other trial designs which do not require randomization such as matched pair design (198.1).

d) T In a single blind study the subject does not know whether the trial or the control agent is being administered. This reduces any bias (198.1).

e) F In a double blind study neither the subject nor the observer knows the nature of the drug administered so reducing bias (198.1).

199 There is a lag period in MCQ questions between clinical introduction of a drug and its first appearance in the examination. The corresponding lag period for vivas can be extremely short and questions may be asked before a drug reaches clinical use. It is important to keep up with current literature.

The following statements are true of ketorolac:
a) maximum plasma concentrations after intramuscular injection are seen in one hour
b) may be given by both oral and parenteral routes
c) is highly protein bound
d) has potent anti-inflammatory effects
e) may increase the bleeding time

200 The final question in the pharmacology section returns to home. Alfentanil is a companion to us all and has rapidly achieved a high degree of popularity amongst the opioid family.

Alfentanil:
a) has a shorter duration of action than fentanyl
b) is metabolized to noralfentanil
c) is less potent than fentanyl
d) has a pKa of 7.4
e) has a short half life due to a low volume of distribution

References
199.1 BJA (1990) 55   p 445–447
200.1 Dundee, Clarke & McCaughey   p 219–220

199a) T After i.m. administration of ketorolac maximum plasma concentrations are seen in 45–60 min (199.1)
   b) T Ketorolac is unusual among the NSAIDs because it may be given by oral, and i.m. routes (199.1). The drug obviously has great potential.
   c) T Ketorolac is highly protein bound (199.1). This is generally true of the NSAIDs as a group.
   d) F In contrast to the potent analgesic activity, ketorolac has minimal anti-inflammatory actions (199.1).
   e) T Ketorolac increases the bleeding time but as yet this appears to be of little clinical significance (199.1).

200a) T Alfentanil has a much shorter duration of clinical effect than fentanyl. In UK practice it is the most evanescent opioid available. The terminal half life is very short at 1.5 h (200.1).
   b) T In common with fentanyl the major route of metabolism is oxidative *N*-dealkalation. This process yields noralfentanil (200.1).
   b) T Alfentanil has approximately one third to one fifth the potency of fentanyl. This fact is borne out by the relative doses of each drug necessary for a clinical effect (200.1).
   d) F The pKa of alfentanil lies below the plasma pH at 6.8. That is unusual and results in a high proportion of the drug being unionized in the plasma. This helps provide a quick onset of action (200.1).
   e) T Alfentanil is a good example of drug engineering. Changing the molecule of fentanyl deliberately to reduce volume of distribution was successful in producing an agent which has a rapid onset and offset of action (200.1).

201 The adrenal cortex secretes two groups of hormones. The mineral-ocorticoids are so called because of their role in the regulation of extracellular fluid composition. The glucocorticoids, named on account of their involvement with blood glucose concentration, comprise the second group.

Glucocorticoids:
a) show a circadian rhythm with maximum plasma levels around midnight
b) have secretion that is regulated principally by negative feedback to the anterior pituitary
c) inhibit the reaction between antibody and antigen
d) may cause lymphopenia
e) may mask the symptoms if given to patients with bacterial infection

202 The production of hyperglycaemia by hormones may be the result of their primary physiological action or a lesser effect of hormones whose main activity is distinct from glucose regulation. In the completions below there are examples of both mechanisms.

Hormones producing hyperglycaemia include:
a) growth hormone
b) prolactin
c) glucagon
d) thyroid hormone
e) oestrogen

References	
201.1 Ganong	p 346–353
202.1 Guyton	p 823–824
202.2 Harper	p 481–482
202.3 Ganong	p 326–328
202.4 Data Sheet Compendium	p 536
202.5 Data Sheet Compendium	p 1057

201a) F Circadian or diurnal rhythm is a feature of glucocorticoids but the maximal secretion is seen in the early morning before waking. If the day is artificially prolonged then the adrenal cycle is also prolonged. The biological clock that controls the rhythm is located in the suprachiasmic nuclei of the hypothalamus (201.1).

b) T Glucocorticoids inhibit ACTH secretion. The degree of anterior pituitary inhibition is a linear function of glucocorticoid levels. Note that inhibition also occurs at hypothalamic level. Inhibition is due to an action on DNA and takes several hours to develop (201.1).

c) F Glucocorticoids do not affect the combination of antigen with antibody and have no effects on histamine once it is released *but* they do prevent histamine release (201.1).

d) T Glucocorticoid hormones reduce the circulating lymphocyte count and lymph node size. Glucocorticoids inhibit production of interleukin-2 by T lymphocytes so stopping lymphocyte proliferation (201.1).

e) T Febrile reaction, toxicity, and other symptoms may be completely suppressed by glucocorticoids with potentially lethal consequences (201.1). Remember the effect of glucocorticoids in masking the signs of acute abdomen.

202a) T Cellular uptake and utilization of glucose are reduced by growth hormone, causing an increase in blood glucose. This may rise as high as 50–100% above normal (202.1).

b) T Prolactin stimulates growth hormone-like metabolic changes. Hyperglycaemia is a result of reduced peripheral utilization of glucose and enhanced hepatic production of glucose via gluconeogenesis (202.2).

c) T Glucagon is glycogenolytic, gluconeogenic, lipolytic, and ketogenic. Glucagon will bind to hepatic cell receptors, activate adenylate cyclase, and increase intracellular cAMP. The resulting activation of phosphorylase by cAMP increases breakdown of glycogen and so increases blood glucose (202.3).

d) T Thyroxine raises blood sugar and may upset the control of diabetic patients (202.4).

e) T Glucose intolerance is a feature of oestrogen-containing preparations (202.5).

203 This question stays within the metabolic arena and will severely test your knowledge of glucose metabolism. So great a degree of complexity in the completions will not be encountered frequently.

Glucose:
a) enters red cells by diffusion along a concentration gradient
b) is actively co-transported across small intestinal mucosa in association with sodium ions
c) does not permeate freely through capillary endothelium except in the liver
d) a falling plasma concentration causes release of glucose from muscle glycogen into the plasma
e) enters glomerular filtrate from the blood plasma by a passive process

204 Starvation tests knowledge of metabolism and its changes under extreme conditions. The metabolic response to starvation makes a good revision companion to the subjects of metabolic response to surgery and trauma. It is not easy to find detailed material to revise. Lehninger (204.1) is recommended reading.

In starvation:
a) muscle glycogen and brain glycogen are replenished by gluconeogenesis
b) free fatty acid oxidation in the liver, muscle, and heart is increased
c) ketone bodies produced in the liver from free fatty acids can be utilized by brain cells but glucose is still essential
d) glucose can be formed from fatty acids
e) the odour of the breath is due to ketosis

References

203.1	Guyton	p 745–746
203.2	Guyton	p 172–173
203.3	Guyton	p 771–772
203.4	Ganong	p 270–271
203.5	Lote	p 46
204.1	Lehninger	p 840–844

203a) F Cell membranes contain pores that allow particles of a maximum molecular weight of 100 Daltons to pass through. Glucose has a molecular weight of 180 Daltons. Glucose is transported through membranes by protein carrier molecules in a process called facilitated diffusion (203.1).

b) T In the gastrointestinal membrane and renal tubule, glucose is transported by the mechanism of active sodium co-transport. Active transport of sodium provides energy for transporting glucose <u>against</u> a concentration gradient (203.1).

c) T In the standard capillary (e.g. muscle) the capillary permeability for glucose is 0.6 times that for water (203.2). Hepatic sinuses are extremely permeable compared with other capillaries despite a similar endothelium (203.3).

d) F Glycogen can be broken down in the liver to increase blood glucose. The kidneys can also contribute to an increase in blood glucose by metabolizing glycogen. The glucose-6-phosphatase present in these organs is the enzyme for conversion of the glucose-6-phosphate from glycogen to glucose. When adenylate cyclase is stimulated in the muscle by adrenaline, the activation of phosphorylase that occurs does cause a breakdown of glycogen. The glucose that is formed in the skeletal muscle is catabolized in the muscle itself and causes a rise in blood lactate level (203.4).

e) T In the glomerulus there is free passage of molecules with a molecular weight of less than 7000 Daltons. The concentration of glucose in the glomerular filtrate matches that in the plasma water. Glucose is mainly reabsorbed in the proximal tubule (203.5).

204a) F The brain does not contain glycogen and usually relies on glucose from the blood for its energy supply. Gluconeogenesis is the term for glucose production (204.1).

b) T Free fatty acids can be oxidized in the liver to produce ketones that are used for energy by the brain. Alternatively they can be oxidized in heart, kidney or muscle to produce energy (204.1).

c) F In starvation a ketone, beta-hydroxybutyrate, is produced in the liver from free fatty acids and this can be used by the brain cells instead of (or in addition to) glucose (204.1).

d) F No glucose can be formed from fatty acids by mammals (204.1). This is a species dependent ability.

e) T Ketone bodies are formed and these impart the characteristic odour to the breath (204.1).

205 The phraseology of MCQ questions can be a vexed subject. In the following question the nub is what is meant by 'moderate exercise'. If you have no idea of the definition do not attempt it before reading the reference section.

In moderate exercise from rest:
a) cerebral blood flow will increase
b) heart rate will increase by less than 40 beats/min
c) an oxygen debt will occur
d) P_{CO_2} will fall by about 1 kPa
e) mixed venous oxygen content will fall

206 Both the eye and the ear are potential topics. Although the sense organs are not frequently featured in the examination they are included here for completeness of coverage.

With respect to the eye:
a) the optic disc contains CSF
b) the superior rectus muscle is supplied by the trochlear nerve
c) the intraocular pressure is 16 mmHg
d) the Edinger–Westphal nucleus is involved in accommodation
e) the macula has the highest density of rods

References

205.1 Nunn	p 297–299
205.2 Berne & Levy	p 562
205.3 Ganong	p 531
205.4 Guyton	p 946–947
206.1 Guyton	p 683
206.2 Guyton	p 565
206.3 Guyton	p 543–544
206.4 Ganong	p 142
206.5 Ganong	p 137

205a) F Moderate exercise is defined as being <u>below the subject's anae-robic threshold</u> and the arterial blood lactate is not raised. The subject is able to transport all the oxygen required and this corresponds to work levels up to about 100 W (205.1). Despite changes in blood pressure (a rise in systolic, diastolic, and pulse pressure) the cerebral blood flow remains constant throughout a period of moderate exercise (205.2).

b) F If moderate exercise is defined as less than 100 W or 600 kg/m min^{-1} then the heart rate will increase from 64 beats/min to 122 beats/min approximately (205.3).

c) F According to the definition of moderate exercise this is below the anaerobic threshold. No lactate will be released into the circulation and no oxygen debt will occur (205.1).

d) F Blood gas results remain nearly normal even during severe exercise. Respiration is stimulated by neurogenic mechanisms, not by changes in blood gases (205.4).

e) T The arterial oxygen content cannot be increased but cardiac output and extraction at tissue level increase to achieve an increase in oxygen flux. Cardiac output increases less than extraction and so the mixed venous oxygen content will fall (205.1).

206a) F The dura mater of the brain extends as a sheath around the optic nerve and blends with the sclera of the eye. When pressure rises in the cerebrospinal fluid system it also rises in the optic nerve sheath. This pressure impedes flow in the retinal vein so producing retinal oedema (papilloedema) as the optic disc is more distensible than the sheath (206.1).

b) F The superior rectus muscle is supplied by the third cranial or oculomotor nerve and is responsible for moving the eye in an upward direction (206.2).

c) T Aqueous humor is being continually formed and reabsorbed. It is the balance between these two processes that determines the intraocular pressure. Formation is by the ciliary body in a similar manner to the production of CSF by the choroid plexus, and absorption is via the canal of Schlemm. The pressure, which may be measured by tonometry, ranges between 12 and 20 mmHg (206.3).

d) F The Edinger–Westphal nucleus is part of the response to light but is not involved in the mechanism of accommodation (206.4).

e) F The macula lutea is a pigmented spot at the posterior pole of the eye and is also called the fovea centralis. It is a rod-free portion of the retina with densely packed cones and no overlying blood vessels. Cones are responsible for high acuity colour vision in bright light (206.5).

207 The electrophysiology of nerve and muscle is complex. Be careful to get the ionic concentrations the correct way round when considering the generation of the action potential. It is easy to become confused and lose marks.

The action potential:
a) is generated by differing ionic concentrations of sodium and potassium
b) a negative potential inside the nerve drives potassium ions to the outside
c) depolarization is caused by the transfer of sodium ions across the membrane
d) in the resting state the potential inside the nerve fibre is +85 mV
e) at the peak of the action potential the voltage change is 35 mV

208 Questions based on the electrocardiogram are common. It can prove difficult to revise the topic but there are specific texts on the interpretation of ECGs which can supplement the usual general physiology textbooks.

The T wave of the ECG occurs:
a) at the beginning of the refractory period
b) during atrial systole
c) during ventricular diastole
d) during repolarization of the ventricle
e) at the time of the first heart sound

References	
207.1 Ganong	p 47–51
207.2 Guyton	p 51–66
208.1 Guyton	p 101–102

207a) T The ionic fluxes of sodium and potassium form the basis of the action potential. The initial decrease in membrane potential causes potassium efflux. When depolarization exceeds 7 mV the sodium channels open and influx of sodium occurs (207.1).

b) F Potassium moves out of the cell down its concentration gradient despite being actively transported into the cell (207.1).

c) F The initial depolarization is not caused by sodium influx. Note that initial depolarization is caused by increased potassium *efflux*. When the depolarization caused by this effect reaches 7 mV a voltage-dependent effect opens the sodium channels. Be careful with this one (207.1).

d) F The inside potential of neurones is always negative. In the resting state the correct figure is –90 mV (207.1).

e) F The voltage change which occurs at the peak of the action potential is 125 mV (207.2). The change here is taken to refer to the swing from resting potential.

208a) F The T wave occurs in the late phase of ventricular contraction at the start of ventricular repolarization which is the point when the ventricular fibres start to relax (208.1).

b) F Atrial systole occurs just after the P wave (208.1).

c) F The T wave occurs just prior to the end of ventricular systole (208.1).

d) T The T wave occurs at the start of ventricular repolarization which is just before the end of ventricular systole. This is detailed above (208.2).

e) F Dangerous! The T wave will normally approximate to the timing of the second heart sound (208.2).

209 It appears as though some of the following completions are based on anatomy. The structure of the lung is, however, intimately related to its function. Respiratory physiology includes morphology.

The following statements are true of alveoli:
a) the mean wall thickness is 5 μ
b) the pores of Kohn connect to bronchioles
c) they have a mean diameter of 0.4 mm at FRC
d) type I cells produce surfactant
e) half bud directly from alveolar ducts

210 This is deliberately grouped together with the preceding question to emphasize the importance of the morphology of the respiratory tree.

With regard to the tracheobronchial tree:
a) Weibel's classification has 26 generations
b) maximum resistance to gas flow is seen in the eighth generation
c) flow related collapse may lead to trapping
d) respiratory bronchioles take part in gas exchange
e) peak inspiratory flow rate is 400 l/min

References	
209.1 Nunn	p 10–13
209.2 Nunn	p 16–18
210.1 Nunn	p 6–12
210.2 Nunn	p 58–62
210.3 Dunnill & Colvin	p 124

209a) F The wall thickness of alveoli, although very variable, is a great deal less than 5 μ. A figure of 0.4 μ is quoted (209.1). The mean figure for the number of alveoli is a staggering 300 million.

b) T The pores of Kohn are fenestrations in the alveolar septa which allow collateral ventilation between air spaces. Connections have been described between small bronchioles and their related alveoli (209.1).

c) F The mean diameter of alveoli at FRC is 0.2 mm. In 1731 Reverend Stephan Hales estimated this figure to be 1/100 inch (209.1).

d) F It is the alveolar epithelial type II cells that produce and store surfactant (209.3). Other cellular contents of the alveoli includes type III brush cells, alveolar macrophages, mast cells, non-ciliated bronchiolar epithelial cells, and APUD (amine precursor uptake and decarboxylation) cells.

e) T Half of all alveoli do arise directly from alveolar ducts (209.1).

210a) F Weibel's classification has 23 generations (210.1). These extend from generation zero, which is the trachea, to generation 23 which comprises the alveolar sacs.

b) F The contribution of airways beyond the eighth generation to airway resistance is small. This is because their aggregate cross sectional area is comparatively large (210.1). *remains up to 7th generation*

c) T Flow related collapse of airways occurs when the normal trans-mural pressure gradient is reversed, usually during expiration. Flow related collapse is common in emphysema when trapping of air will occur (210.2).

d) T This is as obvious as their name suggests (210.1). Respiratory bronchioles take part in gas exchange.

e) F Expiratory flow rate is higher than inspiratory. Peak inspiratory flow rate is 300 l/min adults (210.3) whereas peak expiratory flow rate is 400 l/min.

211 It is rare for a Part 2 FRCAnaes MCQ paper to exclude chemoreceptors. The differences between the central and peripheral chemoreceptors should be clearly understood.

The peripheral chemoreceptors:
a) are stimulated by a reduction in the content of oxygen in arterial blood
b) contain dopamine
c) affect the adrenal
d) are stimulated by exercise
e) are supplied by the glossopharyngeal nerve

212 Different factors affect the two classes of chemoreceptor although some stimuli cause an equal response from both.

The central chemoreceptors:
a) are stimulated by hypoxia
b) are related to the inferior cerebellar artery
c) are the major source of the response to hypercapnia
d) are stimulated by ascent to high altitude
e) are affected by CSF bicarbonate concentration

References	
211.1 Nunn	p 81–85
212.1 Nunn	p 85–89

211a) F The peripheral chemoreceptors are fast responding monitors of arterial blood which respond to Po_2, Pco_2 and H^+ *or* a drop in their perfusion. Reduced content of oxygen does not stimulate the peripheral chemoreceptors provided that the Po_2 stays normal (211.1).

b) T The peripheral chemoreceptor is synonymous with the carotid body. The glomus cells therein contain dopamine which is known to alter chemoreceptor sensitivity (211.1).

c) T Adrenal secretion is influenced by the peripheral chemoreceptors. Other effects of chemoreceptor stimulation include bradycardia, hypertension, and an increase in bronchial tone (211.1).

d) T The hyperventilation caused by exercise will result in stimulation of the peripheral chemoreceptors (211.1). The mechanism of this is thought to be the venous/arterial Pco_2 difference which increases in exercise. The central chemoreceptors are too slow to respond in this situation.

e) T The glomus type I cells are in synaptic contact with the glossopharyngeal nerve (211.1).

212a) F The central chemoreceptors are not stimulated by hypoxia whereas the peripheral chemoreceptors are. Central respiratory neurones are depressed by hypoxia and this may result in apnoea (212.1).

b) T The central chemoreceptors are crossed by the anterior inferior cerebellar arteries. The chemosensitive areas lie within 0.2 mm of the anterolateral surfaces of the medulla. These areas are also close to the origins of the glossopharyngeal and vagus nerves (212.1).

c) T Central chemoreceptors contribute 80% or so of the total response to hypercapnia which is mediated by changes in CSF pH (212.1).

d) T The early response to altitude causes a shift in CSF bicarbonate. This stimulates the central chemoreceptors (212.1).

e) T Central chemoreceptors respond to a change in CSF pH. The blood–brain barrier is permeable to carbon dioxide but not hydrogen ions or bicarbonate. Carbon dioxide crosses the blood–brain barrier and hydrates to carbonic acid which then ionizes to produce a pH change. The pH change is inversely proportional to the log of the Pco_2. Changes in CSF bicarbonate occur as a compensatory mechanism to changes in CSF pH by passive distribution across the blood–brain barrier. Active ion transfer may also occur (212.1).

213 The field of respiratory physiology covers a very large area and extensive sections can be tested in a single stem. It is necessary to refer to specialist texts in this subject as the chapters in standard physiology texts will often prove inadequate.

In a normal person:
a) the Pa_{CO_2} rises by up to 1 kPa (7.5 mmHg) during sleep
b) the relationship between alveolar ventilation and alveolar P_{CO_2} is linear up to a P_{CO_2} of 10.7 kPa (80 mmHg)
c) during exercise the increase in ventilation is due to a rise in Pa_{CO_2}
d) metabolic acidosis depresses the CO_2 ventilation response curve
e) peak ventilatory effect occurs when Pa_{CO_2} is 13 kPa (100 mmHg).

214 Dead space is a perennial subject. Learn the definitions of both anatomical and physiological dead space and be able to put values on them. Do not forget to revise techniques for the measurement of dead space.

In a fit adult person, anatomical dead space:
a) increases with increasing lung volumes
b) decreases with hypoventilation
c) is least when the neck is flexed and chin is down
d) may be measured by Fowler's method
e) requires measurement of Pv_{O_2} to be calculated by Bohr's method

References	
213.1 Nunn	p 304
213.2 Nunn	p 111
213.3 Nunn	p 89–91
213.4 Nunn	p 301
214.1 Nunn	p 160–166
214.2 Nunn	p 178

213a) F Tidal volume falls with deepening levels of Non-REM sleep and decreases further during REM sleep. Respiratory frequency increases in all stages of sleep but minute volume decreases in parallel with tidal volume. Arterial P_{CO_2} is usually slightly elevated by about 0.4 kPa (3 mmHg) (213.1).

b) F The key to this question is the word 'alveolar'. The relationship between alveolar P_{CO_2} and alveolar ventilation is hyperbolic (213.2). It is the <u>arterial</u> P_{CO_2} ventilation response curve that is linear up to a P_{aCO_2} of 10.7 kPa (213.3).

c) F During exercise, with oxygen consumption of less than 3 l/min, there is no significant change in either P_{CO_2} or P_{O_2} of arterial blood. Arterial blood gas tensions cannot explain the increase of ventilation during exercise (213.4). Other factors must thus apply.

d) F In metabolic acidosis the CO_2–ventilation–response curve is moved to the left (213.3). There is therefore an increase in ventilation for any given CO_2 and for a given O_2 the gradient of the curve remains the same. This does not constitute depression of response.

e) F When P_{CO_2} rises above 10.7 kPa the linear relationship between P_{CO_2} and ventilation is lost. As P_{CO_2} rises further a point of maximal ventilatory stimulation is reached between 13.3 and 26.6 kPa (213.3).

214a) T The volume of air passages is a function of lung volume. There is an increase in the order of 20 ml in anatomical dead space for each litre increase in lung volume (214.1).

b) T The reduction in dead space is probably due to two factors. Firstly there is a tendency towards laminar flow as hypoventilation occurs so reducing 'functional anatomical dead space'. Secondly, there is a mixing effect of the heartbeat which tends to mix all gas below the carina during hypoventilation (214.1).

c) T The position of the neck and jaw has a pronounced effect on the anatomical dead space. It is minimal with the neck flexed and chin depressed (e.g. 73 ml in adults) and maximal with the neck extended and jaw protruded (e.g. 143 ml in adults) (214.1).

d) T Fowler's method uses carbon dioxide as a tracer gas and measures for this at the lips using a continuous carbon dioxide analyser (214.2).

e) F Bohr's mixing equation is used to calculate the physiological dead space. P_{vO_2} is not a required measurement for this equation which is based on tidal volume and CO_2 (214.1).

215 On meeting a question based on the fetal circulation and the changes that occur in it at birth make a sketch and work from it to clarify the situation.

In the fetus:
a) blood can flow from the vena cava to the descending aorta without passing through the left atrium or left ventricle
b) blood from the ductus arteriosus is more saturated than blood from the ductus venosus
c) the foramen ovale closes as a result of pressure reversal between left atrium and right atrium
d) transition from fetal to adult circulation results from a decrease in pulmonary artery pressure
e) the ductus arteriosus normally closes within 1 hour of birth

216 Severe exercise may be defined as exercise well above the anaerobic threshold accompanied by a rise in blood lactate. This work rate cannot be maintained for very long.

In a healthy subject the response to severe exercise includes:
a) a decrease in stroke volume
b) a decrease in effective blood volume
c) an increase in circulation time
d) a decrease in A–V oxygen difference
e) an increase in the concentration of plasma lactate

References

215.1 Nunn	p 342–344
215.2 West	p 143
215.3 Guyton	p 932–933
216.1 Nunn	p 297
216.2 Berne & Levy	p 564
216.3 Ganong	p 538–539

215a) T Blood can flow from the vena cava through the right atrium, the right ventricle, and then via the pulmonary artery and ductus arteriosus to the descending aorta (215.1).

b) F Blood in the ductus venosus has travelled directly from the placenta so it will have the highest saturation (and Po_2 3.9 kPa). Blood in the ductus arteriosus is mixed with blood returning from the body via the inferior vena cava and superior vena cava and has a lower saturation (and Po_2 2.5 kPa) (215.2).

c) T At birth, as a result of the increase in pulmonary blood flow and a reduction in pulmonary vascular resistance, left atrial pressure rises and the flap-like foramen ovale quickly closes (215.1).

d) T Following the first few breaths there is a dramatic fall in pulmonary vascular resistance with a corresponding decrease in pulmonary artery pressure (215.1).

e) F The changes of pressures between the pulmonary artery and aorta result in a backwards flow within a few hours. Also within a few hours the muscular wall of the ductus starts to constrict the orifice. Within 1–8 days a functional closure has occurred and all flow has ceased. During the following 4 months the ductus arteriosus becomes anatomically closed by the growth of fibrous tissue (215.3).

216a) T Severe exercise is well above the anaerobic threshold and the arterial blood lactate rises. This is an unsteady state and work at this level cannot be maintained. The final result is exhaustion (216.1). With severe exhaustion, the compensatory mechanisms begin to fail. Stroke volume reaches a plateau and often decreases as severe exercise continues (216.2).

b) F Although dehydration occurs, other compensatory mechanisms result in a slight increase in blood volume. Any vasodilator activity on cutaneous vessels is superseded by sympathetic vasoconstrictor activity which increases the effective blood volume slightly (216.2).

c) F The velocity of the circulation can be measured clinically by injecting a bile salt preparation into an arm vein and timing the first appearance of the bitter taste it produces. This is the arm–brain circulation time. With increasing exercise the cardiac output increases and arm–tongue or arm–brain circulation time will fall accordingly (216.3).

d) F The arterial to mixed venous oxygen content difference is markedly increased in heavy exercise because oxygen extraction at the tissues increases dramatically (216.2).

e) T The increase in plasma lactate is embodied in the definition of severe exercise (216.1). Both tissue and blood pH decrease as a result of increased lactic acid and CO_2 production. It is the acidosis which probably determines tolerance levels of severe exercise as it can produce muscle pains, a subjective feeling of exhaustion, and an inability or loss of will to continue (216.2).

217 The determinants of myocardial oxygen consumption are logical. This is one situation where the application of basic principles will help.

Myocardial oxygen consumption:
a) at standstill is 2 ml/100 g min^{-1}
b) is higher than skeletal muscle
c) is determined by endomural wall tension
d) is determined by the contractility of the myocardium
e) is determined by heart rate

218 The determinants of end diastolic volume resemble the determinants of cardiac output. There is an intimate relationship between end diastolic volume and stroke volume.

The following factors increase end diastolic volume:
a) increased venous tone
b) positive intrathoracic pressure
c) atrial systole
d) reduced circulating blood volume
e) reduced ventricular compliance

References
217.1 Ganong   p 531–532
217.2 Berne & Levy   p 564–565

218.1 Ganong   p 528–529

217a) T The level of basal myocardial oxygen consumption during stand-still is determined by causing cardiac standstill and maintaining the coronary circulation artificially. Basal oxygen consumption is 2 ml/100 g min^{-1} and oxygen consumption of the beating heart under basal conditions is 9 ml/100 g min^{-1} (217.1). Be very careful of the term 'basal' as it can be used to describe the heart in standstill or beating but at rest!

b) T The basal oxygen consumption is considerably higher than that of skeletal muscle at rest. A level of 2 ml/100 g min^{-1} is six or seven times greater than that for resting skeletal muscle (217.2).

c) T The determinants of myocardial oxygen consumption are primarily the intramyocardial tension, the contractile state of the myocardium, and the heart rate (217.1). The intramyocardial tension is the tension developed in the muscle of the ventricular wall.

d) T The contractile state of the myocardium, or contractility, is one of the determinants of myocardial oxygen consumption (217.1).

e) T Heart rate is a major determinant of myocardial oxygen consumption (217.1).

218a) T Increased venous return raises preload; an increase in preload will cause a rise in end diastolic volume (218.1).

b) F Positive intrathoracic pressure will tend to reduce preload by impeding venous return and thus lead to a reduced end diastolic volume (218.1).

c) T Atrial systole aids ventricular filling so increasing end diastolic volume (218.1).

d) F A reduction of circulating volume reduces end diastolic volume (218.1). This is a classic situation of a reduction in preloading.

e) F A reduction in the compliance of the ventricle reduces the end diastolic volume (218.1). Compliance is reduced as the ventricle becomes 'stiffer' and thus less distensible.

219 The function of the sense organs forms part of the scope of physiology. The eye and the ear will not be frequently encountered in the examination. See Question 206.

With respect to the ear:
a) the membranous labyrinth is surrounded by perilymph
b) the organ of Corti is the organ of hearing
c) neurons from the cochlea terminate in the pons
d) the crista ampullaris is located in the semicircular canals
e) auditory information from both ears reaches the superior olive

220 A question on the nose completes the coverage on sense organs and may provide some light relief. Not essential revision, however.

With respect to the nose:
a) olfactory receptors only respond to chemicals in contact with the mucous membrane
b) activated receptors cause an increase in cyclic AMP
c) there are no pain fibres in the nose
d) adaptation occurs
e) the smell pathway ends in the olfactory cortex

References	
219.1 Ganong	p 158–164
220.1 Ganong	p 171–174

219a) T The inner ear is made of two sections, the bony labyrinth in which lies the membranous labyrinth (which is surrounded by perilymph) (219.1).

b) T The organ of Corti is located on the basilar membrane. It is the organ that contains hair cells which are the auditory receptors (219.1).

c) F The termination of the cochlear division of the vestibulocochlear acoustic nerve is in the dorsal and ventral cochlear nuclei of the medulla oblongata (219.1).

d) T The crista ampullaris is the receptor for balance and it is located in each of three semicircular canals in each ear (219.1).

e) T From the cochlea a variety of paths run via the inferior colliculi and medial geniculate bodies to the auditory cortex. The information from both ears reaches each superior olive (219.1).

220a) T This is the basis of the mechanism of smell. Chemicals must be dissolved in the layer of mucous overlying the membrane before a 'smell' is detected (220.1).

b) T Cyclic AMP binds to sodium channels and the resultant influx of sodium produces a receptor potential (220.1).

c) F There are exposed nerve endings in the nose which act as nociceptors. These endings are branches of trigeminal pain fibres and are responsible for initiating sneezing, lachrymation, and respiratory inhibition as a reflex response to nasal irritants (220.1).

d) T Repeated stimuli result in lesser degrees of perception for that specific stimulus. The threshold for other odours remains unchanged. Adaptation is mediated both centrally and at receptor level (220.1).

e) T The pathway passes in a posterior direction, from the cribriform plate through the intermediate olfactory stria and lateral olfactory stria to the olfactory cortex. The olfactory cortex is part of the limbic system (220.1). Remember pheromones.

221 The physiology of neuromuscular transmission and neuromuscular function has great clinical relevance. Frequent opportunities exist for viva questions. A favourite concerns the effect of each type of muscle relaxant on the 'train of four'.

With respect to the neuromuscular junction:
a) the synaptic cleft is 10 nm wide
b) acetylcholinesterase is freely distributed in the extracellular fluid of the synaptic cleft
c) the rapid influx of sodium and calcium to the interior of the cell produces the action potential
d) fatigue will not occur
e) the end plate is insulated from surrounding fluids

222 The mixed bag of completions makes for a searching question. The topic is loosely based on nerve and muscle physiology. In the examination be prepared to draw the reflex arc.

The following statements are true:
a) intrafusal and extrafusal fibres are found in the muscle spindle
b) the knee jerk reflex is the only monosynaptic reflex in the human
c) in the stretch reflex the central synapse neurotransmitter is glutamate
d) a monosynaptic reflex can be modified by occlusion
e) the Bell–Magendie law applies to the spinal cord

References

221.1 Guyton	p 80–83
222.1 Ganong	p 115–116

221a) F The synaptic cleft is 20–30 nm wide and is occupied by a basal lamina (221.1). This is composed of a thin layer of reticular fibres which permits the diffusion of extracellular fluid.

b) F The enzyme acetylcholinesterase is attached to the matrix of the basal lamina in large quantities (221.1). It is this enzyme which is responsible for the rapid destruction of acetylcholine when released into the synaptic cleft.

c) F From a 'practical point of view' only sodium ions flow through the ionic channels because the extracellular concentration of calcium ions is less than one fiftieth of the concentration of sodium ions (221.1). Note that in theory the ionic channels are large enough to allow positive ions through.

d) F Under usual conditions fatigue of the neuromuscular junction will only occur at the most exhausting levels of activity. Artificial stimulation at 100 Hz for several minutes will, however, cause fatigue (221.1).

e) T The entire area of the neuromuscular junction is covered by one or more Schwann cells. These will act to insulate it from surrounding fluids (221.1).

222a) F Extrafusal fibres are the fibres of the regular contractile muscle whereas intrafusal fibres are the more embryonal fibres of the muscle spindle (222.1).

b) F The knee jerk reflex is the most commonly quoted monosynaptic stretch reflex. However, there are many others which should not be forgotten, such as the ankle jerk, elbow jerk, and the masseter stretch reflex (221.1).

c) T Glutamate is the central neurotransmitter which has a role in the stretch reflex (222.1).

d) T Both monosynaptic and polysynaptic reflexes can be modified by spatial and temporal facilitation, occlusion, subliminal fringe effects, and also sundry other effects (222.1).

e) T The principle that in the spinal cord the dorsal roots are sensory and the ventral roots are motor is known as the Bell–Magendie law (222.1).

223 The muscle spindle and its associated physiology can be bewildering. The nervous pathways involved in the gamma system should be clear in your mind before attempting this question.

The following statements apply to the gamma motor system:
a) gamma fibres are a subgroup of group A fibres
b) gamma efferent fibres only terminate on the nuclear bag fibres
c) the gamma efferent system is excited primarily by the bulbo-reticular facilitatory region
d) gamma efferents allow separate spindle responses to phasic and tonic events
e) stimulation of the gamma efferent system results in impulses in Ia fibres

224 The morphology of muscle sheds light on the physiological process of contraction. Diagrams of the contractile mechanism are easy to find. The relevant section in 'Gray's Anatomy' is useful (224.2).

With regard to myosin and actin:
a) a myosin molecule has a molecular weight of 480 000 Daltons
b) myosin heads form cross bridges with actin filaments
c) the myosin head can act as an ATPase enzyme
d) actin filaments are inserted in Z discs
e) ADP molecules are the active sites on actin filaments

References

223.1 Guyton   p 591
223.2 Guyton   p 592–597
223.3 Ganong   p 118–119

224.1 Guyton   p 70–72
224.2 Gray's Anatomy   p 545–562

223a) T A-gamma fibres (5 μ diameter) transmit pulses to the intrafusal fibres of the muscle spindles. A-alpha fibres (10–20 μ diameter) transmit pulses to the extrafusal fibres of the skeletal muscle (223.1).

b) F Dynamic gamma motor fibres terminate on the nuclear bag cell. Static gamma fibres terminate on both nuclear bag fibres and nuclear chain fibres (223.1).

c) T The gamma motor system is excited firstly by the bulboreticular facilitatory region of the brain stem and secondarily by impulses transmitted into this area from the cerebellum, basal ganglia, and cerebral cortex (223.2).

d) T Dynamic efferent stimulation increases muscle spindle response to phasic events, and static efferents increase spindle responses to tonic events (223.3).

e) T Stimulation of gamma efferents causes the contractile ends of the intrafusal fibres to shorten, therefore stretching the nuclear bag portion of the spindles. This initiates impulses in the Ia fibres via the annulospiral endings (223.3).

224a) T The myosin filament is made up of myosin molecules each having a molecular weight 480 000 Daltons (224.1).

b) T It is the myosin heads that attach to the actin filaments and rotate to produce the sliding filament mechanism for muscle contraction (224.1).

c) T The myosin head acts as an ATPase to cleave ATP. The energy that results from cleaving the high energy phosphate bond energizes the contraction process (224.1).

d) T The bases of the actin filaments are very firmly inserted into the Z discs while the other ends protrude in both directions into the sarcomeres to lie in the gaps between the myosin molecules (224.1). The morphology of the muscle is clearly displayed in 'Gray's Anatomy' (224.2).

e) T The ADP molecules are the active sites on the actin filaments that react with the cross bridges of myosin (224.1).

225 The liver is an organ of great diversity. Apart from the functions of the liver (see Question 64) micro structure, macro structure, and determinants of liver blood flow may appear in questions.

The following statements apply to liver blood flow:
a) the liver receives blood from both systemic and portal circulations
b) it comprises 30% of cardiac output
c) it is 1500 ml/min
d) regulation is by local factors
e) regulation is by the parasympathetic nervous system

226 It would seem entirely appropriate to juxtapose a question on the liver with one on bilirubin. Apart from bilirubin metabolism and excretion the topic also encompasses the formation of bilirubin from haemoglobin breakdown.

With regard to bilirubin:
a) it is protein bound
b) bilirubin diglucuronide is less water soluble than bilirubin
c) it is responsible for the colour of bile
d) conjugated bilirubin is absorbed from the gut
e) urobilinogen is formed from bilirubin

References
225.1 Guyton   p 771–772
225.2 Current Anaesthesia and Critical Care
           (1990) 1.4   p 196–203
226.1 Ganong   p 467–468

225a) T The liver receives approximately 1100 ml/min flow from the portal sinusoids. In addition the hepatic artery supplies systemic blood (225.1) at a rate of 350 ml/min or so. The total blood flow is thus in the order of 1450 ml/min from both these sources, varying between 1100 and 1800 ml/min (225.2).

b) T The total flow from both portal and systemic sources is approximately one third of the cardiac output (225.1). The importance of the hepatic arterial supply should be emphasized because this supplies oxygen to the connective tissue and the walls of the bile ducts.

c) T The systemic contribution to liver blood flow is about 350 ml/min (225.1).

d) T Local metabolic factors play a role in the regulation (225.1). Such factors are very important in the regulation of the hepatic arterial input. In general, liver blood flow is maintained at a constant rate by a variety of mechanisms in line with its importance as an organ.

e) F It is the sympathetic nervous system which is involved and it is principally the storage areas of the liver which are under nervous control (225.1). The liver has a considerable capacity as a storage organ and is very distensible.

226a) T In the circulation bilirubin is bound to albumin (226.1). Not all bilirubin is tightly bound and most can dissociate in the liver where it is free to enter the liver cells after which it binds to cytoplasmic proteins.

b) F Bilirubin is conjugated with glucuronide to render it more water soluble and thus to aid excretion by the kidney (226.2). Glucuronyl transferase is the enzyme responsible for this process and this is located on smooth endoplasmic reticulum.

c) T This is no trick! Not all answers are difficult. Bilirubin and biliverdin give bile its unique yellow–green colour (226.1). Urobilinogens do not share this coloration.

d) F Conjugated bilirubin is poorly absorbed from the gastrointestinal tract in sharp contrast to the unconjugated form (226.1).

e) T The action of gut flora causes the formation of urobilinogens (which are colourless compounds) from bilirubin (226.1).

227 The metabolism of fat and protein is of lesser importance than carbohydrate metabolism. It is desirable to have a working knowledge of the transport, utilization, and storage of fats and proteins as a minimum.

The following statements apply to fat:
a) triglycerides are the major dietary source
b) fat is stored in muscle
c) it is absorbed into intestinal lymphatics
d) it provides energy
e) fat may be absorbed directly into portal blood

228 In a similar style the emphasis moves on to protein metabolism. Be wary of completions containing numerical values for absorption such as d).

The following statements apply to protein:
a) digestion begins in the mouth
b) absorption of amino acids is rapid in the ileum
c) it is subject to active absorption
d) 10% of ingested protein enters the colon
e) it provides energy

References	
227.1 Guyton	p 728
227.2 Guyton	p 755–756
227.3 Guyton	p 734
227.4 Ganong	p 293
227.5 Guyton	p 734
228.1 Guyton	p 727–728
228.2 Ganong	p 293

227a) T Most ingested fat is in the form of triglycerides (227.1). These are neutral fats which consist of a glycerol nucleus and three associated fatty acids.

b) F Only in pathological conditions is muscle a site of fat deposition. Normally this will not occur, fat being stored mainly in two tissues — adipose tissue and the liver (227.2).

c) T The absorption of fat is complex and involves both direct diffusion into the brush border and ferrying by bile acids. Monoglycerides and free fatty acids are soluble in chyme and in this form they are able to diffuse easily through the epithelial membrane of the brush border. After transport triglycerides are reconstituted within the cells of the brush border (227.3) in smooth endoplasmic reticulum.

d) T Fat is a dietary energy source. The calorific yield amounts to 9 cal/g. This is more than twice that of protein and carbohydrate (227.4).

e) T Fat absorption into the portal blood only holds true for small quantities of short chain fatty acids (227.5), for example those contained in butter fat.

228a) F The digestion of protein begins in the stomach (228.1). The enzyme pepsin begins the process and requires an acid medium. This is provided by the secretion of hydrochloric acid by the parietal cells of the stomach.

b) F Absorption of amino acids is rapid in the duodenum and jejunum but slow in the ileum (228.1). Although information on the precise mechanism of absorption is limited, at least four separate carrier systems exist.

c) T There is an active transport mechanism from lumen to mucosal cell involving simultaneous sodium transport. This is the so-called sodium co-transport system which applies equally to the absorption of glucose (228.1).

d) F Usually only 2% or so of ingested protein escapes absorption before reaching the colon (228.1).

e) T Protein is an obvious dietary source of energy yielding around 4 cal/g (228.2).

229 The respiratory physiology of the cough and sneeze is very similar with one fundamental difference. A group of responses which is associated includes vomiting and swallowing. This group is beloved of examiners in physiology.

Coughing:
a) is a reflex action
b) consists of a forced expiration against a closed glottis
c) may create intrapleural pressures over 100 mmHg
d) can generate air velocity of 600 mph
e) is integrated in the pons

230 Sneeze is a less well known process than cough although the two share some common features. Some completions below will be obvious but take care with the more obscure ones.

Sneezing:
a) is integrated in the medulla oblongata
b) occurs in response to irritation of the nasal mucosa
c) is a forced expiration against a closed glottis
d) results from signals in the seventh cranial nerve
e) is preceded by deep inspiration

References
229.1 Ganong   p 629–630
229.2 Ganong   p 214

230.1 Ganong   p 214

229a) T Coughing is a reflex action which occurs in response to irritation of the airway. The purpose of coughing is to keep the airway clear. A voluntary cough is also possible (229.1).

b) T This is exactly the basis of cough in contrast to sneezing when the glottis remains open during the forced expiration (229.1). The basis of cough is a deep inspiration followed by a forced expiration against a closed glottis. When the glottis is suddenly opened the intrapleural pressure is released producing high velocity outflow of air.

c) T Such high intrapleural pressures can lead to problems, pneumothorax for example (229.1).

d) T A surprisingly high speed! This explains the very good clearing effect of coughing on both secretions and foreign bodies (229.1).

e) F The reflex of coughing is integrated in the medulla oblongata and not the pons (229.2). The medulla is the integrating centre for several reflexes including swallowing, sneezing, gagging, and vomiting.

230a) T The integration of the sneezing reflex is very similar to that for coughing and occurs in the medulla oblongata (230.1).

b) T This is a very obvious true answer. Some marks may be had easily after all! (230.1).

c) F In sneezing the expiration takes place through an open glottis (229.1). This is the fundamental difference between the process of cough and sneeze.

d) F Signals from the nasal mucosa travel in the fifth (trigeminal) nerve (230.1). The seventh cranial nerve is the facial.

e) T In exactly the same manner as for coughing the deep inspiration which will normally amount to a vital capacity breath is necessary to generate the explosive outflow of gas (229.1).

231 Opioid physiology has been advancing at breakneck speed since Hughes and Kosterlitz published their paper in 1975. An area of great interest to practising anaesthetists, it should be studied in detail. It is difficult to keep up to date but a review in the BJA (231.2) is informative.

With respect to opioid peptides:
a) pro-opiomelanocortin is found in the anterior lobe of the pituitary gland
b) beta endorphin is the natural ligand of mu receptors
c) pro-opiomelanocortin produces MSH
d) pro-opiomelanocortin produces ACTH
e) prepro and pro forms exist

232 Along with the knowledge of the structure and function of the opioid peptides came detailed information on receptors and their roles.

The following associations are found:
a) mu receptors and dysphoria
b) kappa receptors and calcium channels
c) delta receptors and respiratory depression
d) kappa receptors and diuresis
e) mu receptors and delta receptors

References
231.1 Ganong   p 99
231.2 BJA (1991) 66   p 370–380
232.1 BJA (1991) 66   p 370–380

231a) T Pro-opiomelanocortin is a large precursor molecule to the opioid peptides which is found in the anterior lobe of the pituitary gland (231.1). Within the structure of this molecule lie the amino acid sequences of several other physiological fragments, one of which is ACTH.

b) T Beta endorphin is the probable natural endogenous ligand for mu receptors. Exogenous agonists at these receptors embrace most of the commonly used opioid analgesics which exert their analgesic effects via mu receptors (231.2).

c) T The sequence of the precursor contains the sequences of both melanocyte-stimulating hormone (MSH) and ACTH which are formed after release by the process of peptide cleavage (231.1).

d) T The structure of this large molecule is interesting. It contains many separate amino acid sequences including gamma MSH, ACTH, and beta lipotrophic hormone (231.1).

e) T The opioid peptides have several precursors and these include both pro and prepro forms (231.1).

232a) F Mu receptors are associated primarily with supraspinal analgesia. They have not been implicated in dysphoria (232.1).

b) T Kappa receptors are coupled with calcium channels and have little affinity for either mu or delta agonists (231.2). In common with the mu population it has been suggested that there are two subtypes of kappa receptor. Most of the products of prodynorphin react with kappa receptors. One kappa ligand has been linked to sexual behaviour although the significance of this is not known. Kappa receptors also mediate spinal analgesia via dynorphin pathways (232.1).

c) T Delta and mu receptors have both been implicated in the mechanism of respiratory depression (232.1). It is still not entirely certain that these two exist as separate entities. Certainly it would seem that mu and delta receptors cannot coexist in the same cells.

d) T In contrast to mu, kappa receptors are involved in diuresis (232.1). It is thought that mu receptors are responsible for the anti-diuretic effect of most opioids.

e) T Mu receptors are definitely associated with delta receptors and the debate goes on as to whether the two types are interconvertible depending on local ionic conditions. This was postulated some years ago by Bowen and Gentleman. Recently Pleuvry aired the view that mu and delta may correspond to mu_1 and mu_2 isoreceptors (232.1). Both mu and delta receptors are coupled to potassium channels in contrast to the calcium role of the kappa receptor.

233 The measurement of glomerular filtration rate must not be confused with renal plasma flow. A distinction needs to be made between the use of inulin and para-aminohippuric acid (PAH) for these measurements.

The following are desirable features in a substance suitable for the measurement of GFR:
a) tubular reabsorption
b) no metabolism
c) no effect on GFR
d) free filtration
e) non-toxic

234 Clearance appears regularly in the examination. The concept must be clearly understood. A definition of clearance is desirable if not essential.

The following statements apply to clearance:
a) it is defined as the amount of plasma cleared of a substance in one minute
b) it may be calculated by the formula:

$$\frac{\text{quantity of urine (ml/min)} \times \text{concentration in urine}}{\text{concentration in plasma}}$$

c) inulin clearance measures GFR
d) PAH clearance measures RPF
e) sodium has a clearance of one

References	
233.1 Ganong	p 655–656
233.2 Anaesthesia Review 7	p 67–74
234.1 Guyton	p 306–307

233a) F The ideal substance for measuring GFR should neither be re-absorbed nor secreted by the tubules in order to achieve an accurate value (233.1). Glomerular filtration rate should be measured using a substance that is freely filtered by the glomeruli in addition to the above conditions. The amount of such a substance in the urine per unit of time must have been obtained by filtering the volume of plasma that contained this amount of the substance. For an update on tests of renal function refer to Anaesthesia Review 7 (233.2).

b) T Metabolism would give a falsely high value for GFR (233.1) since a lower urinary concentration will result.

c) T This is obvious otherwise a nonsensical value for GFR will be obtained (233.1).

d) T The substance which most closely meets these criteria, although not absolutely ideal, is inulin which is a polymer of fructose found in nature in dahlia tubers (233.1).

e) T Otherwise patient compliance would be rather low! (233.1).

234a) T This is the usual definition of clearance (234.1). Often discussion occurs around the concept of clearance which is well illustrated by this definition.

b) T This is the formula which is used (234.1). Conceptually this is in complete accord with the above definition. The most common application of this principle that we meet in practice is endogenous creatinine clearance which may be measured by the application of the formula.

c) T Inulin (molecular weight 52 000 Daltons) is the substance which most closely resembles the ideal for measurement of GFR (234.1).

d) T Para-aminohippuric acid, in common with inulin, is able to pass across the glomerular membrane but PAH is secreted into the tubules and is thus used to estimate renal plasma flow (RPF) (234.1).

e) T A figure of 0.9 is most often quoted (234.1). This is close enough to a value of 1 to qualify for a 'true' response.

235 If you find these two questions on simple biochemistry anything but elementary then you are not prepared to sit this examination. Osmolality and osmolarity have different definitions and different units. They are not interchangeable concepts.

With regard to osmolality:
a) units are mosmol/l of solvent
b) normal plasma value is 290 mosmol/l
c) it can be calculated from the sum of the plasma ionic components
d) it is a measure of oncotic pressure
e) plasma proteins make up a large part

236 Extracellular fluid is featured here but the completions could be used with respect to intracellular or interstitial fluid equally well.

The extracellular fluid:
a) volume may be measured with inulin
b) volume may be measured with mannitol
c) comprises 50% of body weight
d) is 20 litres in the adult
e) is more difficult to measure than intracellular fluid

References
235.1 Aitkenhead & Smith   p 286–287
235.2 Dunnill & Colvin   p 74

236.1 Ganong   p 2–3

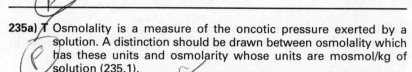

235a) T Osmolality is a measure of the oncotic pressure exerted by a solution. A distinction should be drawn between osmolality which has these units and osmolarity whose units are mosmol/kg of solution (235.1).

b) T Normal plasma osmolality falls within the range 280–300 mosmol/L (235.2).

c) F An estimate of osmolality can be obtained from twice sodium plus twice potassium plus urea plus glucose (plasma values) (235.1). Whilst not completely accurate this is a useful rule of thumb.

d) T Osmolality is a measure of colloid oncotic pressure of the plasma (235.1).

e) F Plasma proteins contribute very little to osmolality (235.1).

236a) T Radioactive [^{14}C] inulin is the most accurate way of estimating extracellular fluid (ECF) volume (236.1). ECF volume is not easy to measure. That is largely because the limits are poorly defined and few substances are completely extracellular. Mannitol and sucrose have been used but give less reliable results than inulin.

b) T Mannitol may be used but will not give an accurate value as it is not totally extracellular in distribution (236.1).

c) F ECF comprises 20% of body-weight (236.1). This value represents about 14 litres in a standard 70 kg adult male of which 3.5 litres is in plasma and 10.5 litres interstitial.

d) F ECF comprises 14 litres in the adult (236.1). See above for detail on the compartments.

e) F Intracellular fluid volume cannot be directly measured and therefore has to be estimated by subtracting ECF from total body water (236.1). As such the measurement suffers from the inaccuracies which beset each of these estimates themselves.

237 Comprehending the physiology underlying the concept of tubular maximum provides the key to elucidating the handling of solutes by the kidney.

The tubular maximum for glucose:
a) is relatively independent of endocrine function
b) is dependent on blood glucose
c) is 375 mg/min
d) is primarily dependent on the number of functional nephrons
e) is not homogeneous between nephrons

238 Mixed venous oxygen concentration yields an estimate of overall oxygen consumption from all organs. Each organ has its own extraction related to metabolic need.

Venous oxygen content from the following organs is less than that of mixed venous blood:
a) heart muscle
b) skin
c) kidney
d) liver
e) brain

References	
237.1 Lote	p 58–60
238.1 Ganong	p 562–563

237a) T This is generally true although there is a limit of blood sugar of about 20 mmol/l over which the tubular maximum for glucose (Tm_G) is inadequate to ensure reabsorption of the glucose load (237.1).

b) F The tubular maximum is independent of blood glucose (237.1) but note the comment above to the effect that this will only hold true for values up to 20 mmol/l.

c) T The value of tubular maximum for glucose is 380 mg/min or so (237.1). This is a mean of the tubule population all of which have differing values. See below.

d) F Each nephron has its own tubular maximum. This value is not exactly the same for each which leads to the splay of the glucose excretion curve (237.1).

e) T The variation in tubular maxima between nephrons is marked and represents a degree of inhomogeneity (237.1).

238 The arteriovenous oxygen difference for an organ gives a guide to the metabolic activity per se of that organ. It would thus be expected that the values for cardiac and skeletal muscle would be high along with that for brain. The value for the whole of the body indicates a mean of the figures for each separate organ. This is implicit in the measurement of mixed venous oxygen saturation.

a) T The A–V oxygen difference for cardiac muscle is 114 ml/l as opposed to 46 ml/l for mixed venous blood (238.1).

b) F The A–V difference for skin is 25 ml/l (238.1).

c) F The A–V difference for kidney is 14 ml/l. This represents a low metabolic activity level (238.1).

d) F Liver has an A–V oxygen difference of 34 ml/l (238.1).

e) T The A–V oxygen difference for brain is 62 ml/l reflecting the high metabolic rate of the brain. Muscle also has a relatively high value of 60 ml/l (238.1).

239 While pathways in the central nervous system are important in their own right, particular attention should be paid to the physiology of pain.

With respect to pain transmission:
a) fast pain travels in A delta fibres
b) pain is associated with the ventral spinothalamic tract
c) descending tracts modulate pain transmission
d) the pain gate lies in the substantia gelatinosa
e) slow pain travels in C fibres

240 The embryological development of the four chambered mammalian heart is complex. The sinoatrial and atrioventricular nodes arise from different sides of the embryo. Be certain not to confuse right and left. The remainder of the question involves basic cardiac physiology.

The sinoatrial node:
a) is derived from the right side of the embryo
b) is situated on the wall of the left atrium
c) initiates cardiac excitation
d) has a resting membrane potential of 60 mV
e) has a discharge rate related to temperature

References

239.1 Ganong	p 124–134
239.2 Wall & Melzack	p 1–18
240.1 Ganong	p 504–506

239a) T Fast pain is transmitted in A delta fibres and it is the speed of conduction (12–30 m/s) in these which gives rise to the term 'fast' pain (239.1).

b) F The lateral spinothalamic tract is the major route of pain transmission. The ventral spinothalamic tract carries mainly the touch modality (239.1).

c) T There are several descending modulations which affect pain transmission (239.1).

d) T Gate control of pain transmission has four main elements: afferents, descending control, segmental interactions in the dorsal horn, and transmission cells. Laminae I and II of the dorsal horn are intimately connected with the integration of these elements. Laminae II and III of Rexed are synonymous with the substantia gelatinosa, the site of the original gate postulated by Wall and Melzack (239.2).

e) T Slow pain travels in the C fibres which are unmyelinated and have a diameter of 0.4–1.2 μ. The speed of conduction in these fibres is considerably slower than the A delta route (0.5–2 m/s). Fast and slow transmission of pain results in the initial sharp unpleasant feeling followed by a later duller intense pain. The temporal separation of these two perceptions depends on the distance from the brain of the injury (239.1).

240a) T This statement is true but the atrioventricular (AV) node is derived from the left side of the embryo (240.1). This may help to explain why the adult has predominantly <u>right</u> vagal innervation of the sinoatrial (SA) node and left vagal innervation to the AV node.

b) F The SA node is situated on the wall of the right atrium (240.1) at the junction with the superior vena cava. This generally holds true for four chambered mammalian hearts.

c) T The SA node is a rhythmically discharging focus in which the cells show the property of pacemaker potentials. Spread of depolarization arising in the SA node generates cardiac excitation. Although pacemaker potentials are marked in both SA and AV nodes, other portions of the conducting system show latent pacemaker ability which may supervene in certain pathological states (240.1).

d) F The resting potential of the SA node is minus 60 mV (240.1). If you meet a question like this one make very sure of the <u>minus</u> value before marking it as true.

e) T In a directly related manner—increased firing in pyrexia and vice versa (240.1). This is logical. Consider the bradycardia of hypothermic states.

Bibliography

The bibliography provides the key to the shortened references used throughout the book. The shortened title used in the text forms the first line of each section below and this is followed by the full reference. Where appropriate a weighting on the value of each source for revision has been given. Texts to which the Part 2 FRCAnaes candidate should have constant access are marked with an asterisk (*).

AHFS

McEvoy G K (ed) 1989 American Hospital Formulary Service. American Society of Hospital Pharmacists, Bethesda

Analogous to the British National Formulary. It is not a book worthy of direct study but has useful applications in searching out some of the more minor pharmacological properties which has been its role in this book. Most hospital pharmacies carry this text and it is well known to drug information departments.

Aitkenhead & Smith

Aitkenhead A R, Smith G (eds) 1990 Textbook of anaesthesia, 2nd edn. Churchill Livingstone, Edinburgh

Purposely written for trainees in their first 1–2 years of practice and therefore not a core text for basic science revision. The popularity of the textbook nonetheless makes it very suitable for reference to more clinically biased questions. The outline chapters on physiology and pharmacology are useful for an overall view.

*Anaesthesia

Lunn J N (ed) Anaesthesia (The Journal of the Association of Anaesthetists of Great Britain and Ireland). Academic Press, London

One of the two major UK journals which is sent to every member of the Association of Anaesthetists. Apart from original papers there are a number of review articles which provide good up-to-date revision material.

Anaesthesia Review

Kaufman L (ed) From 1982 Anaesthesia review. Churchill Livingstone, Edinburgh

This excellent series attempts to bridge the gap between original papers appearing in journals and their subsequent distillation into textbooks. It succeeds in this regard well. Each volume contains detailed reviews on a topic with extensive referencing. The series is now up to volume 8. Recommended.

Atkinson, Rushman & Lee

Atkinson R S, Rushman G B, Lee A J 1987 A synopsis of anaesthesia, 10th edn. Wright, Bristol

Synopsis provides very good summarizing notes on the pharmacology of anaesthetic drugs. These sections are very useful as they provide both detailed information on drugs and detailed references.

Bennett

Bennett D H 1989 Cardiac arrhythmias, 3rd edn. Wright, Bristol

Not a book which needs to be studied extensively, Bennett has as its major strength the detailed coverage of current thinking in the diagnosis and management of cardiac arrhythmias.

Berne & Levy

Berne R M, Levy M N (eds) 1988 Physiology. CV Mosby, St Louis

A major physiology text which can be used to augment the role of Ganong and Guyton which will be the books that most candidates used as undergraduates. Berne & Levy has been utilized for its strengths in areas where the major two are a little thin, such as the physiology of exercise.

*BJA

Smith G (ed) British Journal of Anaesthesia. Professional and Scientific Publications, London

BJA resides alongside 'Anaesthesia' as a major UK periodical for the specialty. It also has wide international readership. Now the official journal of the College of Anaesthetists, BJA is immensely valuable as a source of up-to-date knowledge. The review articles and postgraduate issues are excellent.

*BNF

British National Formulary 1991. British Medical Association and The Royal Pharmaceutical Society of Great Britain, London

The BNF is distributed free of charge to practising doctors. It is a useful source of clinical information on all drugs used in this country. Editions are published 6-monthly so references have been made to sections rather than page numbers. The section numbers remain constant to each subject and are given at the top of each page in BNF.

Braunwald

Braunwald E (ed) 1988 Heart disease: a textbook of cardiovascular medicine, 3rd edn. W B Saunders, Philadelphia

A major text covering most cardiovascular topics which provides useful information for Parts 2 and 3 of the anaesthetic diploma. It will be a well-known volume to cardiologists.

*Calvey & Williams

Calvey T N, Williams N F 1991 Principles and practice of pharmacology for anaesthetists, 2nd edn Blackwell Scientific Publications, Oxford

The coverage of Calvey & Williams is not extensive on individual drugs but the great strength of the text lies in the general pharmacology section. Pharmacokinetics is handled particularly well.

Churchill Davidson

Churchill Davidson H C 1984 A practice of anaesthesia, 5th edn. Year Book Medical Publishers, Chicago

A long established textbook of clinical practice which has limited relevance to basic sciences. Nonetheless this volume remains useful for revising clinically related topics.

Concise Oxford English Dictionary

The Concise Oxford English Dictionary 1977 Oxford University Press, Oxford

The language used in multiple choice questions is very exacting. There is no room for error of interpretation hence the use of the OED here.

Current Anaesthesia and Critical Care

Hutton P, Pollard B J, Aitkenhead A R, Simpson P J, Willatts S M (eds) From 1989 Current anaesthesia and critical care. Churchill Livingstone, Edinburgh

This relatively new series contains useful reviews by recognized authors on many aspects of anaesthesia. It is a very important source of information which is more up to date than major texts. The series is designed to build into a reference text over a period. Publication is quarterly and each issue is topic related. Recommended highly.

Data Sheet Compendium

ABPI Data Sheet Compendium 1990–1, Datapharm Publications, London

A collection of data sheets duplicating those found in each box of drugs. The data sheets contain detailed information on each drug. A particular application in revision is the exhaustive list of side effects for each drug. Although revised annually, references to this book should be easy to identify as the compendium is thoroughly indexed.

Datta

Datta S, Ostheimer G W 1987 Common problems in obstetric anesthesia. Year Book Medical Publishers, Chicago

A useful reference source for questions based on the physiology of pregnancy. There is a wealth of clinical obstetric anaesthesia in this text which may well prove useful in the Part 3 examination also. It is difficult to find detailed information on the changes of pregnancy in general physiology texts. This type of book can be used for practice as well as revision and is a sound investment.

Davenport

Davenport H W 1974 The ABC of acid base chemistry, 6th edn. The University of Chicago Press, Chicago

Despite the date of publication, Davenport remains a classic source of wisdom on acid base chemistry. It is included here for that reason alone. Most hospital libraries will have a copy.

Diprivan ®

ICI Pharmaceuticals (UK) 1988 Diprivan®—a versatile intravenous anaesthetic. ICI Pharmaceuticals (UK), Macclesfield

Drug company literature, especially on new drugs, can be a very useful source of data. This publication is well written and informative at a time when the pharmacology of propofol is just filtering through to the major textbooks.

Drugs

Sorkin E M (ed) From 1985 Drugs. ADIS Press, Mairangi Bay, Auckland

A periodical of interest to pharmacists and clinicians containing very detailed papers on selected drugs in each monthly issue. Verification of only one fact has been made from this source which is available in most pharmacy departments.

Drug and Therapeutics Bulletin

Herxheimer A (ed) From 1980 Drug and Therapeutics Bulletin. Consumers' Association, London

A fortnightly periodical from the publishers of 'Which' magazine containing useful reviews and evaluations of drugs. Incorporated with the series are the valuable 'Adverse Drug Reaction Bulletins'.

Dundee, Clarke & McCaughey

Dundee J, Clarke R, McCaughey W 1991 Clinical anaesthetic pharmacology. Churchill Livingstone, Edinburgh

A newly arrived pharmacology textbook from Ireland. Detailed and readable with excellent sections on general pharmacology, this volume has a lot to offer.

Dundee & Wyant

Dundee J W, Wyant G M 1988 Intravenous anaesthesia, 2nd edn. Churchill Livingstone, Edinburgh

Somewhat specialized in content with particular areas of interest, for example the barbiturates.

Dunnill & Colvin

Dunnill R P H, Colvin M P 1989 Clinical and resuscitative data, 4th edn. Blackwell Scientific Publications, Oxford

A useful pocket book for reference throughout your career, packed with factual tables and concisely presented data.

Erikson

Erikson E (ed) 1979 Illustrated handbook in local anaesthesia, 2nd edn. Lloyd Luke, London

A very good text on regional anaesthesia. Erikson also contains a valuable short section on the pharmacology of local anaesthetics. A real classic.

*Ganong

Ganong W F 1989 Review of medical physiology, 14th edn. Appleton Lange, London

Ownership and use of this text is essential for any serious candidate. It is, however, inadequate as a single physiology text for this examination.

Goldschlager & Goldman

Goldschlager N, Goldman M J 1989 Principles of clinical electrocardiography. Lange, London

Useful for revising the ECG; detailed and informative.

*Goodman & Gilman

Goodman, Gilman A, Rall T W, Nies A S, Taylor P 1990 Goodman and Gilman's The pharmacological basis of therapeutics, 8th edn. Pergamon Press, Oxford

Constant reference has been made to this text and it is essential as a pharmacology reference source. Too large for casual reading, the current edition carries on the stout tradition of previous editions. The 8th edition itself refers at times to the 5th!

Gray's Anatomy

Williams P L, Warwick R, Dyson M, Bannister L H (eds) 1989 Gray's anatomy, 37th edn. Churchill Livingstone, Edinburgh

There are very clear, colourful, and helpful descriptions of the morphology of muscle which may be helpful. Obviously the bulk of this volume is anatomy.

*Guyton

Guyton A C 1986 Textbook of medical physiology, 7th edn. W B Saunders, Philadelphia

A useful supplement to Ganong or alternatively a potential main physiology revision text. Guyton is gaining popularity.

Harper

Martin D W, Mayes P A, Rodwell V W, Granner D K 1990 Harper's review of biochemistry, 20th edn. Lange, London

Biochemistry forms part of the basic sciences and Harper is useful particularly for details of human metabolism.

Lancet

The Lancet, The Lancet Ltd, London

One of the two foremost general medical journals in the UK (along with BMJ). Some articles are of direct relevance to anaesthetists.

Lehninger

Lehninger A L 1975 Biochemistry, 2nd edn. Worth Publishers, New York

This is a mighty tome and, although dated, this text continues to be recommended for undergraduate biochemistry in medical schools. There is a very good section on metabolism under stress (for example starvation) and the metabolic response to starvation is covered extremely well. Not for buying perhaps but worth finding a copy to use occasionally.

Lote

Lote C J 1990 Principles of renal physiology, 2nd edn. Chapman & Hall, London

---

Lote is recommended reading for the revision of renal physiology. Pocket sized and readable, it is good value.

Macleod

Macleod J, Munro J 1986 Clinical examination, 7th edn. Churchill Livingstone, Edinburgh

This famous textbook will be known to all medical students. It has been used here for a clinically based question on neurophysiology.

Martindale

Reynolds J E F (ed) 1989 Martindale, the extra pharmacopoeia. The Pharmaceutical Press, London

Another text which is often held by the pharmacy or drug information service. There are times, especially when considering physical properties of drugs, when it may prove invaluable.

Meyler's Side Effects

Dukes M N G (ed) 1988 Meyler's side effects of drugs, an encyclopedia of adverse reactions and interactions. Elsevier, Oxford

The rarer side effects of drugs are featured in this specialized book which is an encyclopaedia of adverse reactions from an international editorial board.

Miller

Miller R D (ed) 1990 Anaesthesia, 3rd edn. Churchill Livingstone, Edinburgh

A large and useful text for all aspects of anaesthetic practice. As this book is American and quite expensive it is not held by all departmental libraries but it is probably the best general textbook available.

Moir

Moir D D 1986 Obstetric anaesthesia and analgesia, 3rd edn. Baillière Tindall, London

There are several specific texts detailing the physiology and pharmacology of pregnancy. Datta and Moir have been used here but there are others, such as Selwyn Crawford, which are equally recommended.

Mollinson

Mollinson P L, Engelfriet C P, Contreras M 1987 Blood transfusion in clinical medicine, 8th edn. Blackwell Scientific Publications, Oxford

A specific source of haematology is vital. This specialized text written for haematologists is helpful.

Nimmo & Smith

Nimmo W S, Smith G 1990 Anaesthesia. Blackwell Scientific Publications, Oxford

Similar in scope to Miller but not quite so comprehensive. Nimmo & Smith is British and may be preferred by trainees for this reason.

*Nunn

Nunn J F 1987 Applied respiratory physiology, 3rd edn. Butterworths, London

No attempt should be made at Part 2 FRCAnaes without previous study of this text. Detailed and comprehensive, Nunn is ideal revision material for respiratory physiology. Highly recommended.

Oxford Textbook of Medicine

Weatherall D J, Ledingham J G G, Warrell D A 1987 Oxford textbook of medicine, 2nd edn. Oxford University Press, Oxford

The OTM is well known as a heavyweight amongst textbooks of medicine. It has been used to supply a few references only.

*Rang & Dale

Rang H P, Dale M M 1991 Pharmacology, 2nd edn Churchill Livingstone, Edinburgh

This textbook of general pharmacology is very comprehensive and well laid out. The limitations of this text are summarized in its own preface: 'this book is intended primarily for preclinical medical students'.

Recent Advances 16

Atkinson R S, Adams A P (eds) 1989 Recent advances in anaesthesia and analgesia 16. Churchill Livingstone, Edinburgh

The 'Recent Advances' and 'Anaesthesia Review' series are important for updating your knowledge especially before vivas. Studying these texts is useful for all three parts of the examination.

Roitt

Roitt I M 1989 Essential immunology, 5th edn. Blackwell Scientific Publications, Oxford

A text that provides a clear, concise approach to immunology. Well established with a large following.

Rowlands

Rowlands D J 1982 Understanding the electrocardiogram. Section 2. Morphological abnormalities. Imperial Chemical Industries, Macclesfield

Sponsored by ICI and published in three parts, there is a great deal of relevant information on the electrocardiogram which makes the series valuable.

Science Data Book

Tennent R M 1976 Science data book. Oliver Boyd, Edinburgh

Most candidates will have a science data book from their school examinations and this is one example. A reference has been made to Tennent for the Greek alphabet!

Scurr, Feldman & Soni

Scurr C, Feldman S, Soni N 1990 Scientific foundations of anaesthesia. The basis of intensive care. Heinemann Medical Books, Oxford

The title of this text suggests that it is *the* book for Part 2 FRCAnaes. Unfortunately, this is far from true due to patchy coverage.

Shoemaker

Shoemaker W C, Thompson W L, Holbrook P R 1984 Textbook of critical care. W B Saunders, Philadelphia

An extensive text of intensive care medicine which is a good reference source for applied cardiovascular physiology.

SOAP

Survey of Anaesthetic Practice 1988. Association of Anaesthetists of Great Britain and Ireland, London

A statement of current anaesthetic practice based on the return of 10 666 questionnaires from around the UK.

Steward

Steward D J 1985 Manual of paediatric anaesthesia, 2nd edn. Churchill Livingstone, Edinburgh

Although intended as a book for clinical use this text has a very good section on the 'foundations of paediatric anaesthesia'. Included are chapters on paediatric physiology, anatomy, and psychology. It has been the source of information for paediatric physiology.

Swinscow

Swinscow T D V 1982 Statistics at square one, 7th edn. British Medical Association, London

A small, concise, and clear text that provides a good starting point for statistics revision.

Trissel

Trissel L A 1990 Handbook on injectable drugs, 6th edn. American Society of Hospital Pharmacists, Houston

A summary of all of the primary published literature on drug stability and the compatibility of injectable drugs used in USA. The wealth of information is difficult to find from any other source.

Tweedle

Tweedle D E F 1982 Metabolic care. Churchill Livingstone, Edinburgh

Not recommended for specific study but contains a wealth of information on metabolism.

*Vickers, Morgan & Spencer

Vickers M D, Morgan M, Spencer P S J 1991 Drugs in anaesthetic practice, 7th edn. Butterworth Heinemann, Oxford

A reliable text on anaesthetic drugs but inadequate as a sole text for the degree and scope of information required for Part 2 FRCAnaes.

Wall & Melzack

Wall P D, Melzack R (eds) 1989 Textbook of pain, 2nd edn. Churchill Livingstone, Edinburgh

A large and detailed textbook from famous editors. Reference has been made to this text in relation to pain pathways and receptors.

*West

West J B 1990 Respiratory physiology — the essentials, 4th edn. Williams & Wilkins, London

A simple overview of respiratory physiology which *must* be supplemented by reference to a more detailed source such as Nunn.

Wintrobe

Wintrobe M M 1981 Clinical haematology, 8th edn. Lea & Febiger, Philadelphia

An extensive haematology textbook which has been used on one occasion only.

Index

The numbers given refer to question numbers rather than page numbers.